first place
4health

leader's guide

Published by Gospel Light
Ventura, California, U.S.A.
www.gospellight.com
Printed in the U.S.A.

Caution: The information contained in this book is intended to be solely for
informational and educational purposes. It is assumed that the First Place 4 Health
participant will consult a medical or health professional before beginning this or any
other weight-loss or physical fitness program.

Library of Congress Cataloging-in-Publication Data
First place 4 health leader's guide.
p. cm.
ISBN 978-0-8307-4525-8 (trade paper)
1. Spiritual life—Christianity—Study and teaching. 2. Spiritual formation—Study and
teaching. 3. Health—Religious aspects—Christianity—Study and teaching. I. Gospel Light
Publications (Firm) II. Title: First Place for health leader's guide.
BV4501.3.F5694 2008
613.2—dc22
2008014954

Rights for publishing this book outside the U.S.A. or in non-English languages are
administered by Gospel Light Worldwide, an international not-for-profit ministry.
For additional information, please visit www.glww.org, email info@glww.org or write
to Gospel Light Worldwide, 1957 Eastman Avenue, Ventura, CA 93003, U.S.A.

contents

foreword

By Carole Lewis
First Place 4 Health National Director

We believe you are embarking on the role of a lifetime by leading a First Place 4 Health class. When I began leading my first class in the fall of 1981, I was a little nervous and unsure of what I needed to do. I wondered if I might have time left over with nothing to say. Well, I worried for nothing. The time spent in that first class literally flew by, and by the end I was wishing for more time, not less.

First Place 4 Health is the most rewarding ministry I have ever been involved in. I have taught Bible study on Sunday mornings, but it seems that people have on their Sunday clothes at our regular church meetings—there just isn't the time to share what is going on in life. The depth of sharing we have in our First Place 4 Health classes is much deeper than I have ever experienced in our Bible study class.

In First Place 4 Health group meetings, we all know coming in that we have something in common with the other members: We all want to have better health and learn how to live a life of balance with Christ in first place. We find a loving group of people who will encourage and pray for us.

As a First Place 4 Health leader, you have the awesome privilege of witnessing lives radically changed as your members learn what it means to give Christ first place in their lives. Your class members will lose weight and learn how to exercise, but I believe the deepest life change occurs as Jesus Christ becomes Lord in their lives. I know this because as I meet people who have had success losing weight in the program, they always tell me the same thing: "I've lost 60 (or however many) pounds in First Place 4 Health, but that's not the most important thing. I've grown closer to God than I ever would have believed."

God is interested in the total person, and for that reason, weight loss may not be the first thing to occur as you lead your members through the group meetings. God may need to work on the spiritual or emotional areas of your members before helping them learn balance in the physical area. Our job as First Place 4 Health leaders is to be there for our members and to encourage them to stay with the class until they receive everything they need to live a life of balance.

The *First Place 4 Health Leader's Guide* will be a rich resource for you as you begin leading your class. Everything you need can be found in the pages of this book. There is also a wealth of information in *Simple Ideas for Healthy Living* that will take you through many sessions of First Place 4 Health. Help is also always available through our website bulletin boards or by contacting another leader or your First Place 4 Health national office staff. Be sure to sign up for our free e-Newsletter and to register your class on our website, www.first place4health.com.

The First Place 4 Health family is the sweetest bunch of folks you will ever meet. I just hope we are all neighbors in heaven!

—Carole

welcome to
first place 4 health!

WHAT IS FIRST PLACE 4 HEALTH?

The First Place 4 Health program is the result of a godly desire placed in the hearts of a group of Christians in Houston, Texas, in 1981. Their desire was to establish a Christ-centered weight-control program. Confident that God had called them to this important work, they began their pursuit with a basic premise: *Because God has saved us from our sins and given us an abundant life, why can't we, as Christians, use that same power in the area of weight control?*

With that in mind, they decided to develop a program that would meet the needs of Christians in the area of weight control. Little did they know what they were undertaking! It was an immense assignment, but knowing that God had called them to the task, they placed all their hopes and aspirations in Him and began the project. They prayed, studied, prayed, read, prayed and wrote—and First Place 4 Health (at that time, simply called "First Place") began to take shape.

Through prayer and study, the First Place founders discerned that in order to be effective, this new program would need to include Scripture reading, prayer, Bible study, Scripture memory, small-group accountability and support, a proven commonsense nutrition plan, exercise and record keeping. They chose Matthew 6:33 as the plan's theme verse because they knew that keeping Christ first in their lives was the key to success in the program: "Seek first his kingdom and his righteousness, and all these things will be given to you as well." Since their aim was for growth in all areas of life—physical, mental, emotional and spiritual—they focused on Jesus' words in Mark 12:30: "Love the Lord your God with all your heart and with all your soul and with all your mind and with all your strength."

These core beliefs remain the foundation of the First Place 4 Health program today. We are convinced that we can only achieve balance in every area of life by putting our relationship with Jesus Christ first, not just in theory, but also in purposeful action that leads to positive transformation.

First Place has always had three underlying themes:

1 **Christ-centered priorities:** Bible study, prayer and Scripture memory

2 **Choices for total health:** addressing the whole person—body, mind, emotions and spirit

3 **Community:** support and accountability through small groups

These three principles are still our core message!

Making the decision to love God with all our heart, soul, mind and strength is just the beginning of the First Place 4 Health journey. The next step is to allow that all-important decision to manifest itself in the way we live our daily lives. That is why we added the words "4 Health" to the First Place name. We felt that it was important to clearly state that giving Christ first place is about healthy, balanced living that involves our body, our mind, our emotions and our spirit.

Meeting weekly in groups of up to 20 people, First Place 4 Health members stay with the same group for the entire 12 weeks. Each meeting includes nutritional information, class discussion, Bible study and prayer. The Live It Plan is based on the USDA Food Guide Pyramid. Using behavior modification techniques, members learn how to be victorious over past eating patterns and to commit their spirit, emotions and mind—and ultimately their body—to God.

The program is designed as three 12-week sessions per year—winter, spring and fall. There are also two six-week Bible studies available for use during the summer break and fall/winter holiday season, or you may decide to do four 12-week sessions. First Place 4 Health is designed to work flexibly with your calendar and location—groups can meet on any day of the week, at any time of day, in a church classroom, a workplace or campus meeting room, a fitness center, or a living room!

WHY CHOOSE FIRST PLACE 4 HEALTH?

A wide variety of people become members of First Place 4 Health, from those who struggle with losing 5 to 10 pounds to those who battle obesity or are tired of yo-yo dieting. Some may join to increase their knowledge about nutrition, to get help with implementing a consistent exercise plan, or to learn how to develop a healthy lifestyle for their family. Whatever their reasons, they soon discover that First Place 4 Health is a biblically based, medically trustworthy wellness program that addresses *the whole person*—physical, mental, emotional and spiritual.

As members are challenged in each area of their lives, they experience *healthiness,* including weight loss and decreased risks of hypertension, heart disease, cancer, diabetes and lower back pain (resulting from a balanced plan of healthy food and exercise). They experience *friendship*—small-group support and accountability, for many people, is a primary ingredient in the recipe for good health. They find *healing* as they uncover and deal with the hurt, anger and fear that are the roots of out-of-control eating. And through Bible study, prayer, and Scripture reading and memorization, they also find *spiritual renewal.*

using the *first place 4 health leader's guide!*

LEADER'S MISSION STATEMENT

The mission of the First Place 4 Health leader is to lead members to put Jesus Christ in first place in their lives by:

- Inspiring them to build godly disciplines into every area of their lives—spiritual, emotional, physical and mental

- Reviving motivation and instilling hope within each member so that he or she, through the Lord's guidance, can make positive behavioral changes

- Providing the member with knowledge about the Live It Plan and other healthy lifestyle information

As a First Place 4 Health leader, you have the opportunity to use your leadership abilities to influence others to put Jesus Christ in first place in their lives. As the Lord works, they will grow spiritually and make progress toward achieving their wellness goals. Transformation comes as group members meet together; share ideas, insights and struggles; affirm and encourage one another; and support one another in prayer. As a leader, you play a vital role in the transformation process.

This *First Place 4 Health Leader's Guide* will help you confidently lead your group in a productive time of learning and genuine community. It is designed to be simple and easy to follow. It is well worth your while to familiarize yourself with its contents—each section has exactly what you need to be a prepared and effective leader. The sections are:

STARTING A FIRST PLACE 4 HEALTH MINISTRY

In this section you will find step-by-step instructions for starting a First Place 4 Health ministry in your church, at your workplace, in your neighborhood or on your campus.

You'll discover how to publicize and promote the new ministry, to conduct an orientation meeting, to organize registration and member materials, to coordinate multiple groups, and much more.

LEADING A FIRST PLACE 4 HEALTH GROUP FOR THE FIRST TIME

Within this section, you will learn everything you need to know about how to guide a group of First Place 4 Health members through each weekly meeting of a 12-week session. You'll also discover information on general leadership principles and ideas for leading a small group effectively. There are lesson plans, outlines, creative meeting ideas and everything else you need to lead your group!

LEADING A FIRST PLACE 4 HEALTH GROUP AGAIN

After you have led your first 12-week session of First Place 4 Health, you'll be ready to tailor your meetings to meet the needs of your group members. This section will give you the tools you need to plan your own lessons and lead your group over the long haul.

ADDITIONAL RESOURCES

This section offers a guide for sharing Christ through First Place 4 Health and listening guides to complete as you watch the *How to Lead with Excellence* DVD. There is also a comprehensive list of resources that we recommend for leaders who desire additional guidance in the area of leadership.

Starting a First Place 4 Health Ministry

getting started!

As you prepare to begin a First Place 4 Health program, we hope that you will consider how this ministry has the potential to radically change the lives of men and women in your community. Though most people join because they need to lose weight or desire better health, a personal relationship with Jesus Christ will change their lives forever.

Consider using First Place 4 Health as an outreach to your community. People needing Christ in their lives are not threatened by coming to a program like First Place 4 Health, as they might be with some other kind of ministry. First Place 4 Health is a welcoming beacon of hope for those God sends our way.

Before you begin making your plans, spend time praying and studying God's Word. God's timing is perfect. Be willing to wait on Him. Be careful about confusing your personal desire for starting First Place 4 Health with what your church, workplace, neighborhood or campus is ready for. There may be a need for First Place 4 Health, but there may not be an interest. Wait for God to open the right doors, and then be ready to move forward when He does!

Make an appointment with your pastor (if you're starting First Place 4 Health in your church), with your employer (if in your workplace) or with whomever can grant permission to proceed. Share information and present materials for their review. Communicate that the First Place 4 Health program is:

- A biblically based and medically trustworthy wellness program

- An outreach tool and a ministry of discipleship

- An annual program divided into four 12-week sessions, with weekly meetings of 1 hour and 15 minutes

If you hope to use meeting space available at your church, workplace or campus, be sure to discuss possible meeting days and times, requirements and expectations for proper care of the facilities, and the availability and cost of childcare. If you want to receive financial support for the ministry to get started, explain that the program is designed to recover any costs initially incurred by the church through member costs.

Give them time to review your proposal and information (don't forget to pray!) and then follow up. When you get the go-ahead, it's time to get to know the First Place 4 Health Group Starter Kit!

inside the group starter kit!

The First Place 4 Health Group Starter Kit includes the following elements:

- *First Place 4 Health* (by Carole Lewis with Marcus Brotherton)
- *First Place 4 Health Leader's Guide*
- *First Place 4 Health Member's Guide*
- *Simple Ideas for Healthy Living*
- *Begin with Christ* Bible study (includes Scripture Memory CD)
- *Food on the Go Pocket Guide*
- *First Place 4 Health Prayer Journal*
- *Orientation and Food Plan* DVD
- *How to Lead with Excellence* DVD
- *Emotions and Eating* DVD
- *Why Should a Christian Be Physically Fit?* DVD
- 25 promotional flyers

(*Note:* While some ministries purchase just one Group Starter Kit for all their groups, many find it difficult to share the various resources—such as the DVDs, which are not available for individual purchase—between multiple leaders. Do what works best for your groups!)

The following is an in-depth explanation of each of the kit's components.

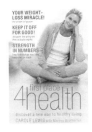

FIRST PLACE 4 HEALTH

This inspiring book by Carole Lewis gives you a behind-the-scenes look at the history and success of First Place 4 Health. You'll find out how the program got started and read the uplifting stories of people who have found balance in their lives through First Place 4 Health. Includes "Before" and "After" pictures, too!

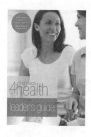

FIRST PLACE 4 HEALTH LEADER'S GUIDE

Whether you decide on a single Group Starter Kit or on multiple kits, a separate *First Place 4 Health Leader's Guide* should be purchased for each group leader—it's the essential reference guide for anyone who wants to lead a First Place 4 Health group.

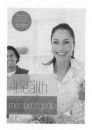

FIRST PLACE 4 HEALTH MEMBER'S GUIDE

This is the go-to guide for everything members need to learn about the First Place 4 Health program and about living a healthy life physically, emotionally, mentally and spiritually. The *Member's Guide* is divided into sections for each of these four areas and walks members step by step through determining a healthy calorie range, seeing the connections between emotions and eating, how to create a fun and effective workout, and much more!

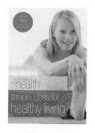

SIMPLE IDEAS FOR HEALTHY LIVING

This handy reference guide contains health tips and information on a wide range of topics that address the four areas of healthy living: body, emotions, mind and spirit. Members can use *Simple Ideas for Healthy Living* to answer questions they may have between group meetings, and leaders will use various topics as part of the Wellness Spotlight in each week's meeting.

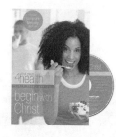

BEGIN WITH CHRIST BIBLE STUDY

Begin with Christ, the first in the series of Bible studies designed specifically to fit with First Place 4 Health's 12-week sessions, includes 12 weeks of personal Bible study, group prayer request forms, a member survey, a personal weight and measurement record, weekly prayer partner forms, Scripture memory verse cards, two weeks of menu plans, a Let's Count Our Miles! excercise chart and a Scripture memory music CD.

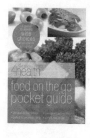

FOOD ON THE GO POCKET GUIDE

A quick and easy reference for eating healthy when eating out. It contains nutrition information for many popular restaurants so that members can make healthy choices even when they're not doing the cooking. And the book's small size makes it perfect for a purse, glove compartment or desk drawer at work.

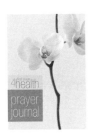

FIRST PLACE 4 HEALTH PRAYER JOURNAL

Journaling is an important part of success in the First Place 4 Health program. Members are encouraged to regularly write their thoughts, feelings and prayers in a journal.

ORIENTATION AND FOOD PLAN DVD

This practical media tool is perfect for introducing those new to First Place 4 Health to the program. It offers basic information about bringing balance to the four-sided person and gives outlines of the Live It Food and Fitness Plans.

HOW TO LEAD WITH EXCELLENCE DVD

First Place 4 Health cares about equipping leaders for their important ministry. This DVD offers general principles about being a great leader, as well as encouragement and practical advice for those who desire to model healthy living through First Place 4 Health.

EMOTIONS AND EATING DVD

Many of us don't eat when we're hungry—we eat when we're sad, angry, lonely or bored! On this invaluable DVD, Cindy Schirle exposes the connection between emotions and eating, and presents helpful ideas for breaking the connection.

WHY SHOULD A CHRISTIAN BE PHYSICALLY FIT? DVD

For nearly 40 years, Dr. Richard Couey has been a professor of Health Sciences at Baylor University, specializing in human anatomy and physiology, nutrition and sports medicine. Now he reveals how eating the proper nutrients can help prevent disease and what the Bible has to say regarding total health.

Once you know the Group Starter Kit inside and out, it's time to introduce the materials to First Place 4 Health group leaders.

recruiting and training
group leaders

LOOKING FOR LEADERS

A potential leader in First Place 4 Health has a desire to minister in the area of wellness and is willing to facilitate a small group. He or she is committed to maturing in the four areas—physical, mental, emotional and spiritual—and is willing to share his or her struggles and successes with others. The best leaders are friendly and communicate easily with others, are able to come early to group meetings (and sometimes stay late!) and are dependable and discreet.

When developing your First Place 4 Health leadership team, we suggest recruiting one leader and one assistant for each group of up to 20 people. These pairs work well when their gifts and strengths are complementary. One leader may be gifted at leading the Bible study discussion and writing notes of encouragement during the week, while the other enjoys facilitating member weigh-in/measurement and evaluating Live It Trackers.

View each member as a potential future leader—once you have at least one group up and running smoothly, you can begin to observe how various people work together. Watch for people in your class who are doing well. Compliment them and ask for their help. It is a natural progression to go from assisting to leading, so look for opportunities to involve your members in some leadership roles.

When recruiting potential leaders, be clear about what is required and give them time to think and pray about making a commitment.

TRAINING AND PREPARING LEADERS

When you have enough group leaders to start your ministry, schedule times for your leadership team to train and prepare together. (If you are starting with one group and you are the leader, we recommend asking someone to assist you, for prayer, support and accountability.) Work through the First Place 4 Health Leader's Guide (each leader should have his or her own copy), focusing on the "Leading a First Place 4 Health Group" section. Also consider watching the *How to Lead with Excellence* DVD and completing the listening guides (see page 119) together.

The goal of training is for group leaders to understand how to facilitate weekly meetings, which include member weigh-in/measurement, Live It Tracker evaluation and Bible study discussion. The goal of preparation is for group leaders to feel confident about their ability to manage group dynamics and discussion. (Read "Preparing to Lead," the introductory chapter in the "Leading a First Place 4 Health Group" section, for more on leading a group effectively.)

When the group leaders in your ministry desire more extensive training, consider some of these options:

- First Place 4 Health workshops are one-day events with basic training for new leaders and creative teaching ideas for experienced leaders.

- First Place 4 Health conferences offer leadership seminars for new and experienced leaders.

- Wellness Weeks provide basic training, inspirational messages and relaxation time for new leaders.

Area meetings, workshops, national conferences and our annual Leadership Summit are all events where First Place 4 Health leaders can come for renewed motivation, education and collaboration. To find out more, call the First Place 4 Health national office or visit the First Place 4 Health website at www.firstplace4health.com.

SUPPORTING LEADERS

If you are the only leader, ask someone in your group to be the person who encourages you and holds you accountable to your weekly weigh-ins/measurements, memory verse recitation and Live It Tracker evaluation. Many times, leaders are selfless to a fault and become burned out quickly for the lack of encouragement and support from another person. To ensure that you lead to the best of your abilities, give adequate attention to yourself and know that you're doing yourself and your group a huge favor!

If you have multiple leaders, organize a leaders' group that meets on a regular basis, such as once a month, for prayer, support and accountability. Area leaders' meetings are also available in some regions. Check the First Place 4 Health website or newsletter for scheduled events.

Now that you have a team of trained and qualified group leaders who are continuing to learn with and support each other, it's time to get the word out about First Place 4 Health!

FREQUENTLY ASKED QUESTIONS

Q: *What about potential leaders who have had gastric bypass surgery?*

A: As weight-loss surgery becomes more common, we will see more and more men and women who have undergone this surgery and want to join First Place 4 Health. But surgery is not a fix-all, and smart members know it. These folks know that they must commit to the program—all facets of it—to maintain whole-person health. It is this commitment that is important when considering a person for leadership in First Place 4 Health.

publicizing and
promoting the ministry!

Before you begin to promote the first session of First Place 4 Health, decide when and where groups will be offered. Consider days and times that are convenient for the group leader(s) and potential members, as well as the need and availability of childcare. Check church, workplace, campus or fitness center calendar for available space for the days/times that work best (you may also investigate the use of facilities such as a community center or an apartment complex clubhouse).

Once you know the *when* and *where* of your First Place 4 Health group(s), work backward and schedule your orientation meeting for two weeks before the first group meeting. Now let potential members know!

WHEN, WHAT AND HOW TO PUBLICIZE

Begin publicity one month before orientation. In each flyer, brochure or announcement, be sure to include:

1 Date, time and location of orientation meeting (it should be made clear that orientation—which presents foundations of the First Place 4 Health program, including the four-sided person and the food plan—is mandatory for new members).

2 Date, time and location of group meeting(s)

3 Contact information (including name, email and phone number) to RSVP for orientation

Not sure how to get the word out? Get creative! Why not design a flyer or brochure to feature on your church's information table or in the Sunday morning bulletin? Set up a display of First Place 4 Health materials in the church foyer so that people can get to know the program. You can also download promotional videos at www.firstplace4health.com to play during the announcement time in a church service or on a small screen as part of a display.

If your groups will meet in a community or fitness center, make sure you post notices at those locations. You could also put up flyers in local businesses and libraries or on campus bulletin boards.

Consider making an announcement in person during the worship service or in adult Sunday School classes (obviously, get permission first!), or on your local television or radio station. Invite a First Place 4 Health member to give his or her testimony, or use the testimonial portion of the *Orientation and Food Plan* DVD in the Group Starter Kit.

Don't forget your local newspaper! Purchasing advertising space is often not as expensive as you might think. Even if you can't afford ad space, it's a good idea to craft a press release and fax it to your local media (see the sample press release on page 27). Be sure to include the contact information for a leader who feels comfortable giving interviews. As an alternative, write your own news article about the program and submit it to your newspaper or community newsletter, as well as to the church office to be included in the church's newsletter and on its website.

Last but not least, be sure to contact previous members—First Place 4 Health alumni— with pre-registration forms by mail or email (see the sample on page 29 or download electronic files from www.firstplace4health.com). Be sure to include information about costs for the upcoming session (see the next chapter!) so that they know exactly what to expect, as well as the dates/times planned for group meetings. Ask them to return their registration form *before* the orientation meeting so that you know exactly how many places are available for new members in each group. The orientation meeting is not required for alumni, but some may choose to come for motivation and inspiration, or to bring a friend who is a potential new member.

FREQUENTLY ASKED QUESTIONS

Q: *We don't have a lot of money. How can we publicize our program to bring in more people?*

A: There are many free avenues available for advertising, including:

- Community newspapers and bulletin boards
- Christian radio announcements
- Flyers in physicians' waiting rooms
- Word-of-mouth advertising
- Members' guests at the end-of-session victory celebration

Sample Church Bulletin Insert

IT'S COMING! DON'T MISS IT!

Do you want to improve your relationships with others? Do you desire to be physically fit? Are you tired of being tired? Would you like to know God in a more intimate way? The answer is coming!

First Place 4 Health, a Christ-centered total-wellness program, will be offered as one of Neighborhood Church's winter discipleship classes. To find out how to achieve emotional, physical, mental and spiritual wellness, visit the First Place 4 Health table in the lobby today!

First Place 4 Health groups will begin meeting the week of January 29 on Mondays from 7:00 P.M. to 8:15 P.M. or on Wednesdays from 9:30 A.M. to 10:45 A.M. To join, attend the orientation meeting on Monday, January 15 at 7:30 P.M. in Room 205. For more information and to RSVP, contact Sue at 555-5555 or sue@neighborhood church.com.

Sample Flyer

YOUR CHANCE TO BE A LOSER!

Losers are winners with First Place 4 Health,
a Christ-centered health and weight-loss program!

Orientation Meeting: Tuesday, June 9,
6:00 P.M. in the Arts & Crafts Room at
Neighborhood Church

Orientation is required for new members.

Six-Week Summer Session:
Group meetings begin June 23 and end August 4.
Groups are offered Tuesdays at noon
and at 7:00 P.M.

For more information and to RSVP,
call Sue at 555-5555
or email sue@neighborhoodchurch.com.

Sample Press Release

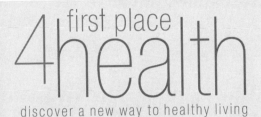

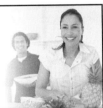

Discover the Most Complete, Christ-Centered Weight-Loss and Healthy Living Program

TO ORDER, CALL 800.4.GOSPEL OR GO TO WWW.GOSPELLIGHT.COM

Neighborhood Church Loses Weight Through Faith-Based Weight Loss Program

FOR IMMEDIATE RELEASE

CONTACT: Sue Smith, Neighborhood Church (555) 555-5555
555 Fifth Street
Houston, TX 77000

Houston, Texas. Every year, Americans spend billions of dollars on weight-loss programs and products. Many are on a search for a quick fix, unwilling to consider permanent changes in their lifestyle as the answer. However, the members of Neighborhood Church have discovered that the Bible holds the answer to the obesity epidemic. By following the First Place 4 Health program, a faith-based weight loss plan supported and endorsed by registered dietitians and physicians, members of Neighborhood Church have already lost a total of 555 pounds.

Meeting in weekly support groups, the members of Neighborhood Church follow a 12-week curriculum that is centered around achieving balance in four essential areas of their lives: emotional, spiritual, mental and physical. First Place 4 Health encourages members to adopt practical disciplines in all four areas. These include regular attendance and fellowship (emotional); prayer, Scripture reading and Bible study (spiritual); Scripture memory and keeping a food record (mental); and eating well and exercising (physical). First Place 4 Health helps members learn how to be victorious over past eating patterns and how to commit their minds and, ultimately, their bodies to God.

I feel better on the inside and look better on the outside than I have in 20 years!
—Jane Doe, who has lost 53 pounds in First Place 4 Health

The First Place 4 Health program has delivered faith-based health and weight management instruction and support to small groups meeting in churches since 1981. First Place 4 Health has been active in more than 12,000 churches with over a half million successful members! The program points members to God's strength and creates a compassionate support group that helps members stay accountable in a positive environment.

At Neighborhood Church, an orientation meeting will be held on Tuesday, June 9, at 6:00 p.m. For more information or to join a First Place 4 Health group, contact Sue Smith at 555-5555.

First Place 4 Health is about more than weight loss—it's about lifestyle change that encourages every participant to find balance in his or her own life.
—Carole Lewis, National Director of First Place 4 Health.

Sample Letter to Alumni

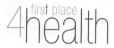

December 18, 2008

Mary Smith
231 Elmwood Ave.
Houston, Texas 77000

Dear Mary,

I'm writing today to invite you to enroll in the winter session of First Place 4 Health hosted by Neighborhood Church. This 12-week session is scheduled to begin the week of January 19 and conclude on April 15, 2009. Group meetings will be held on Tuesdays at 12:00 P.M., Tuesdays at 7:00 P.M., and Wednesdays at 4:45 P.M.

The orientation meeting will be on January 7, 2009, at 7:00 P.M. in the Harbor Room at Neighborhood Church. Because you are an alumnus, it is not necessary for you to attend the orientation, but if you would like to bring a friend who is new to First Place 4 Health, you are welcome to attend.

The alumni registration fee for this session is $40, which includes your copy of this session's Bible study, *Daily Victory, Daily Joy*. Please complete and return the enclosed pre-registration form with your check by January 5, 2009.

Sincerely,

Sue Smith

Sue Smith
First Place 4 Health Director at Neighborhood Church

Sample First Place 4 Health Pre-registration Form

First Place 4 Health
Pre-registration Form

first place
4 health
discover a new way to healthy living

Name _____ ❑ Male
❑ Female
Address _____

City _____ State _____ Zip _____

Phone numbers (H) _____ (W) _____ (Cell) _____

May we call you at work?   ❑ Yes   ❑ No

Email address   _____

Church member?   ❑ Yes ❑ No   If yes, where? _____

Would you like to receive more information about churches in your area?   ❑ Yes ❑ No

If provided, do you need childcare?   ❑ Yes ❑ No

Number of children and ages _____

Friends you wish to be in class with _____

_____

Preferred meeting day _____ Time _____

Leader _____

———————— *DO NOT WRITE BELOW THIS LINE* ————————

Paid   ❑ Yes ❑ No

Amount $ _____ Check # _____ or ❑ Cash

Class assignment day _____ Time _____

Leader _____

Materials received   ❑ Yes ❑ No

member materials and costs

If you plan to make member materials available at orientation, order them at least two weeks prior to the meeting (this requires that you estimate the number of people who will register). If you prefer to wait until you know exactly how many people will register, order materials after orientation, two weeks before the first group meeting.

You can purchase materials at your local Christian bookstore, through Gospel Light (1-800-4-GOSPEL or www.gospellight.com) or from First Place 4 Health (www.firstplace4health.com). If purchasing from your local bookstore, call ahead with your Bible study selection to ensure they order adequate stock before you need them.

MATERIALS

Each *new* group member needs the following:

1 One First Place 4 Health Member's Kit, which includes:

- *First Place 4 Health Member's Guide*
- *First Place 4 Health* by Carole Lewis
- *Simple Ideas for Healthy Living*
- *Food on the Go Pocket Guide*
- *First Place 4 Health Prayer Journal*
- *Emotions and Eating* DVD
- *Why Should a Christian Be Physically Fit?* DVD

2 One First Place 4 Health Bible study, which includes:

- 12 weeks of daily Bible study
- Scripture memory verse CD and cards
- Weekly Prayer Partner forms
- 12 weekly Live It Trackers

- 2 weeks of menu plans, including grocery lists and recipes
- Personal weight and measurement record
- 100-Miles Club exercise record
- "Let's Count Our Miles!" exercise record
- Leader Discussion Guide

The Member's Kit is a one-time purchase and contains everything the individual members in your group need to succeed. Having only the selected Bible study will limit members' success and will make the group meetings more difficult, with some having all of the materials and some having only a few. (For an in-depth breakdown of each of the kit components, read "Inside the Member's Kit" in the next section.)

A married couple or parent/child in the same group might share a Member's Kit, but each should have their own Bible study.

Each *returning* member needs only the First Place 4 Health Bible study selected for the upcoming session.

COSTS

Before orientation, figure out the costs for new and returning members to participate in the upcoming session. Consider charging $10 to $20 more per member than the actual cost of their materials, and then using additional monies to cover such items as:

- Shipping fees
- A reliable scale for weekly weigh-ins
- Tape measures
- Childcare
- The victory celebration
- Fitness testing
- Additional resources (such as books, food models[1] and other instructional items)
- Partial scholarships for those who cannot afford to purchase all member materials
- First Place 4 Health materials for the leader and assistant leader
- Leadership training such as workshops, conferences, the First Place 4 Health annual Leadership Summit and Wellness Weeks

If a potential member wants to join First Place 4 Health but feels that he or she cannot afford the costs, there are several options. You may offer to provide the Bible study while the person purchases the Member's Kit. You may ask people in your group or church to donate toward a partial scholarship. (We do not recommend giving *full* scholarships because we believe that each member needs to invest in order to see a return on their investment.

We also do not recommend a payment plan unless your church is willing to absorb the cost if the member drops out before all payments have been made.)

Now that you know what materials members need, have researched how much those materials cost, and have determined any additional costs for the upcoming session, you are ready to host an orientation meeting and register those potential members!

Note

1. Food models can be purchased online at websites such as www.enasco.com and www.ncescatalog.com.

orientation and registration!

Two weeks before the first group meeting, host an orientation meeting for potential First Place 4 Health members. The goal is to introduce the program and explain how it works, and then register new members for the upcoming 12-week session. Below is everything you need to know to prepare for and host an orientation!

BEFORE THE MEETING

Plan to host 10- to 15-percent more people than you expect to attend the orientation meeting. (You may have less, but it's always smart to be prepared for everyone God brings!) Reserve a large enough space and make sure there is seating for everyone. Secure any necessary equipment, including a TV and DVD player, and a table to display First Place 4 Health materials. If you prefer to give the "Four-Sided Person" presentation yourself rather than viewing it on the *Orientation and Food Plan* DVD, you'll either need equipment to display the PowerPoint presentation (available for download at www.firstplace4health.com) or a whiteboard or flipchart to draw the diagram yourself. You can find an outline of the "Four-Sided Person" presentation on page 36.

Download the "First Place 4 Health at a Glance" information sheet (see page 39) and modify it to fit your information. Also download the First Place 4 Health registration form (see page 40) and make enough copies of both for everyone. (Go to www.firstplace4health.com to download each document.) Make sure you have enough pens or pencils for everyone.

Consider asking one or two First Place 4 Health alumni to share with potential members about how the program has helped them find greater balance in their lives. (If you decide to do so, remind them in advance that their testimonies should last two minutes or less.)

Arrive early to ensure that everything is set up, working properly and ready to go, and to greet people as they come in. Make your "First Place 4 Health at a Glance" information sheets available from the start so that people can begin to get a picture of the program and how it can meet their needs.

When everyone has arrived, you're ready to begin! Below is an outline to follow for your orientation meeting.

ORIENTATION AGENDA

I. **Welcome and Opening Prayer (2 minutes)**
Introduce yourself and ask the attendees to pray with you. There may be nonbelievers in attendance, so be specific with your instructions. (For example: "Let's all bow our heads and close our eyes as I thank God for His presence with us here tonight.")

II. **Introduce First Place 4 Health (2 to 4 minutes)**
Referring the potential members to the "First Place 4 Health at a Glance" info sheet, introduce the program. To supplement the brief info sheet, you can refer to "Welcome to First Place 4 Health" at the beginning of this *Leader's Guide*.

III. **Alumni Testimony (3 to 5 minutes)**
If before the meeting you asked one or two First Place 4 Health alumni to share their stories, ask them to come forward now. Introduce them to the attendees and explain that the alumni will be sharing very briefly about their First Place 4 Health experience.

IV. **View the "Four-Sided Person" and the "Overarching Themes" Presentations (40 minutes)**
View the "Four-Sided Person" and the "Overarching Themes" segments on the *Orientation and Food Plan* DVD. If you choose, you may present the "Four-Sided Person" PowerPoint presentation available at www.firstplace4health.com. If you prefer to use a whiteboard or flipchart, the diagram can easily be drawn as you give the presentation (see page 36 for an outline). If you present the material, view the DVD as you prepare to ensure that you are confident in your grasp of the ideas.

V. **Registration and Cost Information (5 minutes)**
Announce beginning/ending dates of the upcoming session and the days/times of each group. Explain the cost of the materials members will receive. Give details about childcare, if available.

VI. **Questions and Answers (10 minutes)**
Allow time for questions related to the information you have presented. If questions become too long or too personal, offer to meet with that person at the end of the meeting.

VII. **Commitment Time (5 to 10 minutes)**
Lead the group in prayer to ask God for guidance, and then ask potential members to complete their registration forms. Collect registration forms and fees. If some potential members want to join but did not come prepared to pay the fees, give them a deadline and follow up to confirm.

AFTER THE MEETING

Divide registration forms into groups according to the day and time each member prefers. A group of 12 to 20 works best—if the group is too large, shy people have a hard time sharing and are easily overlooked. Prepare a roster for each group. (A group roster form can be found on page 41 or as an electronic file available for download at www.firstplace4health.com. Make a copy of the roster for each group member and distribute the copies to group leaders prior to their first meeting.

If someone completed a registration form but did not pay their fees, follow up with them to make arrangements for payment. If a potential member wants to join but doesn't feel that he or she can afford it, see "Member Materials and Costs" for some ideas on how to help.

Order materials for all members from your local Christian bookstore, from Gospel Light (1-800-4-GOSPEL or www.gospellight.com) or from First Place 4 Health (www.firstplace4 health.com). Distribute all member materials to the group leaders before their first meeting.

FREQUENTLY ASKED QUESTIONS

Q: I'm the only leader. I had 40 people at orientation and they all joined. Help!

A: If you find yourself with a large group and you have not yet trained other group leaders, recruit several members to be team leaders. Divide the large group into two to four smaller teams. Team leaders can weigh/measure the members in their smaller group, evaluate their Live It Trackers and make contact with each person during the week. Group leaders should stay in close communication with their team leaders and keep abreast of notable information, such as who on each team is struggling or creating difficulties. (See "Recruiting and Training Leaders" for ideas about equipping your new leaders-in-training.)

The "Four-Sided Person" Presentation Outline

As you present the information below, draw the four-sided person diagram according to the instructions.

The basis of First Place 4 Health is Matthew 6:33: "Seek first his kingdom and his righteousness, and all these things will be given to you as well."

How can we do that? Jesus gave us the answer in Mark 12:30: "Love the Lord your God with all your heart and with all your soul and with all your mind and with all your strength." The four-sided person illustration is a simple way to visualize these four areas of our lives.

Draw a diamond with "Jesus" at the center.

First, is Jesus at the center of your life? The name "First Place 4 Health" points to the necessity of inviting Jesus to take first place in our lives, above everything else. Only then can we begin to bring the four areas into balance.

Learning to love the Lord with all our soul means that we are willing to set aside time to develop our relationship with Christ.

Add one bar and label it "Soul."

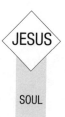

The First Place 4 Health spiritual plan includes spending time with the Lord on a daily basis through Bible study, Scripture reading and prayer. The daily Scripture reading will expose you to the truth of God's Word. In John 8:32, Jesus says that "you will know the truth, and the truth will set you free." During your daily time with Him, the Holy Spirit will reveal truth to you. The Bible study will help you practically apply the truth of God's Word to your life. You will learn how to spend quality time each day with God, and you will grow strong in this area of your life.

We learn to love God will all our heart when we experience genuine community.

Add a second bar and label it "Heart."

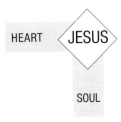

The First Place 4 Health plan for emotional wellness includes a weekly group meeting specifically designed to combat isolation, to provide a loving family of friends, to present information about effective coping techniques, and to promote the truth that you are loved by God. You'll learn the importance of focusing on God and other people rather than on food.

As you reach out to other members of your First Place 4 Health group with intentional acts of encouragement, such as phone calls and emails, you too will be encouraged. Emotional wellness will be one of the greatest benefits you enjoy from learning what it means to give Christ first place in this area of your life. This is done primarily by making attendance to your First Place 4 Health meeting a priority and by encouraging others.

Loving God with all our minds means that we learn a new way of thinking.

Add a third bar and label it "Mind."

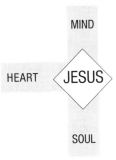

The battle for wellness starts in the mind. The Bible says that God's Word is a divine weapon to help us develop a new way of thinking. Second Corinthians 10:5 says that we can "demolish arguments and every pretension that sets itself up against the knowledge of God, and . . . take captive every thought to make it obedient to Christ." We need to change our minds about a number of things, including the value of exercise, what it means to be full, and how we view ourselves and our bodies.

As a part of this process, you will be asked to memorize one verse of Scripture every week. Scripture memory is a key element that will empower your mind to be transformed, to focus on God and to resist temptation. You will also begin to establish healthy lifestyle habits by keeping a record of your daily choices in a journal, or what we call the "Live It Tracker." Wellness studies show that nothing works better to develop self-awareness and mindfulness.

And finally: You are living in the only physical body you will ever have on this earth.

Add a fourth bar and label it "Strength."

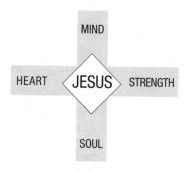

Care of our bodies is an act of stewardship, of caring for a treasure that belongs to Someone else. Properly caring for the gift of our bodies honors our God, who dwells with us through the Holy Spirit. We do this by exercising daily and by choosing quality foods in the appropriate quantities. You will learn how to do both in First Place 4 Health.

This program is about much more than weight loss. The four commitments lead to a well-rounded life in Christ.

- Developing a quiet time will bring you closer to spiritual well-being in an intimate relationship with God.
- The encouragement of others and your weekly meeting will bring emotional support.
- A new way of thinking will be a key element in the transformation God plans for you.
- Exercise and the Live It Plan will give you physical well-being.

The First Place 4 Health materials will help you make positive changes in the way you think and in the way you handle your emotions, in the way you fuel and recharge your body with food and exercise, and in the way you relate to God and others. Are you ready to choose the path of loving God with all your heart, soul, mind and strength? If you take the first step, He will meet you and lead you the rest of the way.

Sample First Place 4 Health at a Glance Information Sheet

WHAT IS FIRST PLACE 4 HEALTH?

The First Place 4 Health program is the result of a godly desire placed in the hearts of a group of Christians in Houston, Texas, in 1981. Their desire was to establish a Christ-centered weight-control program that addressed all areas of life—physical, mental, emotional and spiritual. The resulting program is designed as three 12-week sessions per year—winter, spring and fall. Members stay with the same group for an entire session, encouraging and challenging one another to meet their fitness goals. Each weekly group meeting includes a weigh-in, nutritional information, class discussion, Bible study discussion and prayer. Neighborhood Church is offering groups beginning the week of January 19. Group meetings will be held on Tuesdays at noon, Tuesdays at 7:00 P.M. and Wednesdays at 4:45 P.M.

WHY CHOOSE FIRST PLACE 4 HEALTH?

Maybe you are struggling with losing 5 to 10 pounds or are battling obesity. Perhaps you want to increase your knowledge about nutrition, to get help with implementing a consistent exercise plan or to learn how to develop a healthy lifestyle for your family. Whatever your reasons, you'll soon discover that First Place 4 Health is a biblically based, medically trustworthy wellness program that addresses *the whole person*—physical, mental, emotional and spiritual.

WHAT IS THE COST TO JOIN FIRST PLACE 4 HEALTH?

The cost for your first 12-week session is $140, which includes your First Place 4 Health Member's Kit and the Bible study chosen for this session, *Daily Victory, Daily Joy*. The cost for later sessions is $40.

Sample First Place 4 Health Registration Form

First Place 4 Health
Registration Form

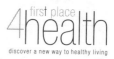

Name _____ ❑ New member ❑ Male

Address _____ ❑ Alumnus   ❑ Female

City _____ State _____ Zip _____

Phone numbers (H) _____ (W) _____ (Cell) _____

May we call you at work?   ❑ Yes ❑ No

Email address   _____

Church member? ❑ Yes ❑ No   If yes, where?

Would you like to receive more information about churches in your area?   ❑ Yes ❑ No

If provided, do you need childcare?   ❑ Yes ❑ No

Number of children and ages _____

Friends you wish to be in class with _____

_____

Preferred meeting day _____ Time _____

Leader _____

———————————— DO NOT WRITE BELOW THIS LINE ————————————

Paid   ❑ Yes ❑ No

Amount $ _____ Check # _____ or ❑ Cash

Class assignment day _____ Time _____

Leader _____

Materials received   ❑ Yes ❑ No

Sample Group Roster

Group Roster

Session Start/End Dates _____ Group Meeting Day _____ Time _____ Leader _____

NAME	ADDRESS (STREET, CITY AND ZIP)	HOME PHONE	WORK PHONE	EMAIL ADDRESS

Leading a First Place 4 Health Group for the First Time

what you need to know about leading a small group!

A s a First Place 4 Health group leader, you have the privilege of teaching others practical knowledge about total health (spiritual, mental, emotional and physical) with enthusiasm and grace. You have been called by God for such a time as this, and we are so thankful for your willingness to serve others and encourage healthy and balanced living in your First Place 4 Health group.

The most important quality in a good leader is *love*. First Corinthians 13 says that we can do all things, know all things or be all things, but if we don't have love, all our efforts are in vain. As you deal with the practical realities of preparing lesson plans and managing group dynamics, ask God to show you how you can do these activities with love, kindness and grace. At the end of the day, your group members won't remember the time you stumbled through the Bible study discussion or when you assigned the wrong Weekly Challenge—but they *will* remember your encouraging words, your kind notes and your supportive hugs.

You will have people in your class who are difficult to love. Yet the ones who need us most are the ones who, many times, are the most unlovely—those who disrupt the group discussion or who never seem to listen to anything we say. These are the ones God has sent us to lead. When you have someone who is hard to love, ask God to love that person through you.

GETTING READY

Don't forget to pray! As you study your lesson plan and gather the materials you need for each week's meeting, pray for each member in your group. Pray that they will be open and receptive to whatever God is trying to do in their hearts and lives, and that God will use you however He chooses in that process.

To prepare the room where you'll hold your group meeting, remember that relationship happens best when it's face to face. If possible, arrange chairs and/or tables in a circle or rectangle so that everyone can see each other. Set up the weigh-in/measurement area away from the main group area, behind a screen or wall, if possible, for privacy.

The time it takes to plan each lesson is time worth spending. Planning will allow you to arrive prepared and with everything you need. The amount of time spent preparing will vary in length depending on your level of experience and learning style. But don't worry! The weekly meeting outlines will greatly assist you in planning for your group meetings.

Collect your materials in advance—there's nothing worse than realizing you've forgotten something when it's too late to do anything about it! If you have an assistant or co-leader, meet with him or her to decide who will take responsibility for each element of the meeting.

When everything is prepared, it's time to lead the group . . .

FREQUENTLY ASKED QUESTIONS

Q: How should I advise a member in my class who has a medical condition?

A: Communicate clearly that whatever recommendations their physician gives should be followed, even if they differ from the general recommendations of First Place 4 Health. The member's medical condition may require very specific and important dietary and exercise instructions, and these are first priority. Be sure they have informed their physician of their involvement with First Place 4 Health. Make an effort to stay informed about any improvement or deterioration of their health.

MAKING IT HAPPEN

Every First Place 4 Health group meeting includes the following elements:

> 15 minutes—Greet and weigh/measure members
> 5 minutes—Discuss previous week's challenge or homework
> 15-25 minutes—Teach Wellness Spotlight(s)
> 20-25 minutes—Bible study discussion (starting Week Two)
> +5-10 minutes—Prayer requests (verbal/written), close in prayer

=1 hour, 15 minutes total

Greet and Weigh Members (15 minutes)

Weigh and measure members (chart on page 61) and listen as they recite the week's Scripture memory verse. (For detailed instructions, see page 57.)

Discuss Previous Week's Challenge and Homework (5 minutes)

Ask your members about the homework and challenge they completed the week before. What did they learn? Were they successful in accomplishing the challenge? Hearing how things are going will help you keep a pulse on the group. Leaders need to *inspect what they expect.* By making time for a brief discussion about weekly assignments, your members will know that you care; this will increase the likelihood that they take their tasks seriously.

Wellness Spotlight (15 to 25 minutes)

For your first 12-week session, each Wellness Spotlight has been prepared for you. (You'll find details in each week's meeting outline.) For later sessions, you can spotlight a wellness issue that specifically concerns your group. *Simple Ideas for Healthy Living* is packed with relevant wellness information to use during this 25-minute period, organized into categories: physical, emotional, mental and spiritual. You can also use segments from one or more of the DVDs included in the Group Starter Kit.

Bible Study Discussion (20 to 25 minutes)

A Leader Discussion Guide is included in the back of each Bible study. Use this guide to lead a discussion about what your members are learning. Try not to lecture. Stimulate discussions by asking open-ended questions. Be cautious not to contribute too much, but try instead to draw out the thoughts and feelings of the members. (To find out more about leading a Bible study discussion, see page 90.)

Prayer Time (5 to 10 minutes)

Don't spend so much time on the Wellness Spotlight and Bible study discussion that you neglect prayer time. Group prayer time is essential to growth and bonding among members. During certain weeks of the session when there is a significant amount of material to cover, ask your group to each choose a member's prayer request form and pray individually after class.

FREQUENTLY ASKED QUESTIONS

Q: *How can I make my group members stick to their commitments?*

A: You can't. People may change their behavior in response to a leader's encouragement, but that does not mean they have changed their core values or beliefs. Values and beliefs are deeply rooted and even spiritual leaders cannot change people; only the Holy Spirit can. Our role as leaders is to encourage our members to listen to and be obedient to how God instructs them. Leaders must encourage encounters with God so that members hear from God directly, not through their leader. Once people hear from God personally, there will be no stopping them from participating in the transforming work of God.

KEEPING IT TOGETHER

Every group meeting will be different: The members (and you!) will have good weeks and bad weeks physically, mentally, emotionally and spiritually. Do your best to plan and prepare, but be flexible. You may plan for an extended time discussing the week's Bible study, but then realize that what is actually needed is an extended time in prayer. Or the discussion may bring up painful memories and emotions for some of your members that need special attention. Be sensitive and responsive to the group's needs.

In group discussions, try to draw out quieter people and limit chattier ones. Don't be afraid to remind the whole group that if there are 12 people and 20 minutes reserved for discussion, each person should speak for less than a minute.

Don't try to be the person with every answer. Don't be afraid to say, "I don't know," "That's a great question" or "Can anyone else help us?" Be yourself. Share your life and your struggles. Let your group see the difference Jesus Christ is making in your life as you strive, as well, to put Him in first place.

Be aware of time during group meetings. Time is important to everyone. We need time to spend time alone with God, with our families, at work and in church activities. Meetings that often go overtime will frustrate many people. By the end of the meeting, members might not be paying attention because they are too busy thinking of what they could—or should—be doing instead. Be sensitive to others by starting and dismissing the meeting on time.

If you need encouragement from other leaders, the First Place 4 Health website is a rich resource. There are bulletin boards where you can connect with leaders all over the globe. Our free monthly e-newsletter is also a great source of information and practical tips for teaching and motivating your members in the four areas (physical, mental, emotional, spiritual).

FREQUENTLY ASKED QUESTIONS

Q: *How do I handle latecomers to the session?*

A: It is best to set a standard from the beginning that no one will be admitted to the group after the second group meeting. If members are allowed to join at any time, bonding with other members will likely be difficult and the progress of the entire group will probably be slowed. Assure any who come later than Week Two that they are welcome to be a part of First Place 4 Health, but for their benefit they need to wait for the next orientation. Help them to locate another group in your area that is starting at a later date, if possible.

first 12-week
session outline!

This is a bird's-eye overview of your group's first 12-week session. When you teach First Place 4 Health for the first time or have a class full of new members, it is extremely important that you follow this outline—it was designed to ensure that each new class receives a clear education about the purpose and scope of the First Place 4 Health program. This teaching plan incorporates all of the fundamental aspects of the program and is organized in an important chronological order. Notice that guidelines on what to teach in your group meeting and what to assign at the conclusion are provided for each of the 12 weeks. There are time estimates for each in-group activity to assist you in efficient planning, and you will also find page references for specific readings or other materials to which you will need to direct your members. You'll find detailed lesson plans for each week in the pages that follow.

WEEK	LESSON PLAN	CHALLENGE AND HOMEWORK
One	1. Greet and weigh/measure members (see "Member Weigh-in/Measurements" on page 57, 15 minutes). 2. Give an overview of the Member's Kit, what members can expect in weekly meetings, and view "The Four-Sided Person" (30 minutes). 3. View the "Grocery Store Tour," the "In the Kitchen with the Dietitian" and the "Using Your Live It Tracker" segments of the *Orientation and Food Plan* DVD. Introduce Live It Step 1: "*Learn* that Change Begins from the Inside Out," (*Member's Guide*, page 102, 30 minutes). 4. Assign homework (2-3 minutes). 5. Prayer (10 minutes).	1. Read "Step 1: *Learn,*" *Member's Guide* page 102. 2. Complete "Your Health Assessment," *Member's Guide* page 112. 3. Complete "Nutrition for Life" to determine a calorie range, *Member's Guide* page 118. 4. Take the Live It Tracker Challenge. 5. Complete Week Two of the Bible study. 6. Memorize this week's Scripture memory verse.

WEEK	LESSON PLAN	CHALLENGE AND HOMEWORK
Two	1. Greet and weigh members (15 minutes). 2. Review and discuss Live It Step 1 (5 minutes). 3. Introduce Live It Step 2: "*Choose* to Set Yourself Up for Success," (*Member's Guide* page 104, 5 minutes). 4. View the "Quiet Time" segment on the *Orientation and Food Plan* DVD (4_2 minutes). 5. Lead Bible study discussion (25 minutes). 6. Assign homework (2-3 minutes). 7. Prayer (10 minutes)	1. Complete "Step 2: *Choose,*" *Member's Guide* page 104. 2. Read "The Nutrition Top 10," *Member's Guide* page 109. 3. Read "The Fitness Top 10," *Member's Guide* page 180. 4. Take the Quiet Time Challenge. 5. Complete Week Three of the Bible study. 6. Memorize this week's Scripture memory verse.
Three	1. Greet and weigh members (15 minutes). 2. Review and discuss Live It Step 2 (5 minutes). 3. Introduce Live It Step 3, "*Use* the Tools Provided in the Live It Plan" (*Member's Guide* page 108, 5 minutes). 4. View "The Nutrition Top 10" segment on the *Orientation and Food Plan* DVD (17 minutes). 5. Lead Bible study discussion (25 minutes). 6. Assign homework (2-3 minutes). 7. Prayer (5 minutes)	1. Complete "Step 3: *Use,*" *Member's Guide* page 108. 2. Read and complete "The Benefits of Physical Activity," *Member's Guide* page 182. 3. View the *Why Should a Christian Be Physically Fit?* DVD. 4. Take the Nutrition Top 10 Challenge. 5. Complete Week Four of the Bible study. 6. Memorize this week's Scripture memory verse.
Four	1. Greet and weigh members (15 minutes). 2. Review and discuss Live It Step 3 (5 minutes). 3. View the "Fitness Top 10" segment on the *Orientation and Food Plan* DVD (6 minutes). 4. Introduce "Grocery Shopping Tips" (*Member's Guide* page 176, 5 minutes). 5. Lead Bible study discussion (25 minutes). 6. Assign homework (2-3 minutes). 7. Prayer (5 minutes)	1. Read "Starting a Basic Exercise Program," *Member's Guide* page 185. 2. Take the Grocery Store Challenge. 3. Take the Fitness Challenge. 4. Complete Week Five of the Bible study. 5. Memorize this week's Scripture memory verse.
Five	1. Greet and weigh members (15 minutes). 2. Discuss the Grocery Store and Fitness Challenges (5 minutes). 3. Review and discuss "The Benefits of Physical Activity" exercise from Week Three (5 minutes). 4. Teach "Understanding the Nutrition Facts Panel" (*Member's Guide* page 149, 15 minutes). 5. Lead Bible study discussion (25 minutes). 6. Assign homework (2-3 minutes). 7. Prayer (5 minutes)	1. Read and complete "The Activity Pyramid," *Member's Guide* page 190. 2. Take the Food Label Challenge. 3. Complete Week Six of the Bible study. 4. Memorize this week's Scripture memory verse.

WEEK	LESSON PLAN	CHALLENGE AND HOMEWORK
Six	1. Greet and weigh members (15 minutes). 2. Discuss the Food Label Challenge (5 minutes). 3. Teach "A Cure for Portion Distortion" (*Member's Guide* page 155, 15 minutes). 4. Lead Bible study discussion (25 minutes). 5. Introduce "Mapping Your Emotional History with Food" (*Member's Guide* page 90, 5 minutes). 6. Assign homework (2-3 minutes). 7. Prayer (5 minutes)	1. View "Emotional Mapping" on the *Emotions and Eating* DVD (all three segments). 2. Take the Emotional Challenge. 3. Complete Week Seven of the Bible study. 4. Memorize this week's Scripture memory verse.
Seven	1. Greet and weigh members (15 minutes). 2. Discuss the Emotional Challenge (5 minutes). 3. Teach "Eating Healthy When Eating Out" (*Member's Guide* page 160, 15 minutes). 4. Discuss "The FITT Formula for Exercise" (*Member's Guide* page 188, 5 minutes). 5. Lead Bible study discussion (25 minutes). 6. Assign homework (2-3 minutes). 7. Prayer (5 minutes)	1. Review and complete "My Prescription for Personal Fitness," *Member's Guide* page 209. 2. Take the Eating Out Challenge. 3. Complete Week Eight of the Bible study. 4. Memorize this week's Scripture memory verse.
Eight	1. Greet and weigh members (15 minutes). 2. Discuss the Eating Out Challenge (5 minutes). 3. Teach "Cardiovascular Exercises" (*Member's Guide* page 193, 15 minutes). 4. Lead Bible study discussion (25 minutes). 5. Assign homework (2-3 minutes). 6. Prayer (5 minutes)	1. Take the Pedometer/Walking/Aerobics Challenge. 2. Complete Week Nine of the Bible study. 3. Memorize this week's Scripture memory verse.
Nine	1. Greet and weigh members (15 minutes). 2. Discuss Pedometer/Walking/Aerobics Challenge (5 minutes). 3. Teach "Strength Training" (*Member's Guide* page 201, 15 minutes). 4. Lead Bible study discussion (25 minutes). 5. Assign homework (2-3 minutes). 6. Prayer (5 minutes)	1. Take the Strength Training Challenge. 2. Complete Week Ten of the Bible study. 3. Memorize this week's Scripture memory verse.
Ten	1. Greet and weigh members (15 minutes) 2. Discuss Strength Training Challenge (5 minutes). 3. Teach "Flexibility and Balance Training" (*Member's Guide* page 205, 15 minutes). 4. Lead Bible study discussion (25 minutes). 5. Assign homework (2-3 minutes). 6. Prayer (10 minutes)	1. Take the Flexibility and Balance Training Challenge. 2. Complete Week Eleven of the Bible study. 3. Memorize this week's Scripture memory verse.

WEEK	LESSON PLAN	CHALLENGE AND HOMEWORK
Eleven	1. Greet and weigh members (15 minutes). 2. Discuss the Flexibility and Balance Training Challenge (5 minutes). 3. Teach "Modifying Recipes" (*Member's Guide* page 165, 15 minutes). 4. Lead Bible study discussion (25 minutes). 5. Assign homework (2-3 minutes). 6. Prayer (10 minutes)	1. Complete Week Twelve of the Bible study. 2. Take the Extreme Recipe Makeover Challenge.
Twelve	1. Greet and weigh members (15 minutes). 2. Discuss the Extreme Recipe Makeover Challenge (10 minutes). 3. Share member testimonies. 4. Celebrate!	1. Take the Maintenance Challenge.

meeting outline!

BEFORE THE MEETING

1. Review this outline and preview the "Grocery Store Tour," "In the Kitchen with the Dietitian" and the "Understanding Your Live It Tracker" segments on the *Orientation and Food Plan* DVD, as well as Live It Step 1 and the Live It Tracker Challenge.

2. Ask for God's wisdom as you follow His direction in leading your group. Pray Hebrews 10:24 for yourself—that you would spur group members on to love and good deeds. Pray for each member by name.

3. Meet with your assistant or co-leader to prepare.
    A. Pray together.
    B. Discuss the Member Weigh-in/Measurements guidelines (pp. 58-60) and fill in the members names on the Weigh-in/Measurement Chart (sample on page 61).
    C. Make a copy of the Group Roster.
    D. Find a basket or a similar container for members to place their Prayer Request Forms (in the back of each member's Bible study) at the beginning of the meeting. At the end of the meeting, each member will draw a request from the basket and pray for that request during the week.
    E. (Optional activity) Arrange with someone to take "Before" pictures of each member at the first meeting. Keep these pictures until the final session to help members see their progress.
    F. Make nametags for everyone in the group. Consider making these permanent rather than disposable.

4. Call members to remind them of the day, time and location of the meeting. If you have already distributed materials, ask them to bring their kit and Bible study to the meeting

and to fill out the Member Survey in the Bible study to turn in. (Have additional Member Surveys on hand at the meeting for any who forget them.) If you have not yet handed out Member's Kits and Bible studies, ask members if they can stay after class for 5 minutes to complete the Member Survey.

   A. If childcare will be available, check with each member to learn how many children will be coming and the children's ages.

   B. If you choose to extend the length of this first meeting, inform members ahead of time.

5. Arrive early to set up the meeting room with chairs and/or tables.

   A. Set up the TV and DVD player, and cue the DVD so that it is ready for viewing during the meeting.

   B. Lay nametags out on a table where members can see them.

   C. Have extra pens or pencils, paper and Bibles available for those who might have forgotten them.

THE MEETING

1. Complete arrival activities (15 minutes).

   A. Greet members.

   B. Place the Group Roster on a table with the nametags and instruct members to check it for accuracy and make corrections if necessary.

   C. Privately weigh/measure each member and record weights and/or measurements on the Weigh-in/Measurements Chart.

   D. (Optional) Take "Before" pictures.

   E. If you have not yet given members their kits and Bible studies, hand out all materials.

2. Open the meeting (15 minutes).

   A. Open in prayer.

   B. Ask group members to introduce themselves. Keep this brief (there will be a "get acquainted" activity for the second meeting).

   C. Briefly walk members through the Member's Kit (see page 62 for an explanation of the contents) and the Bible study. Ask them to fill out the Member Survey, if they have not already done so, and turn it in.

   D. Give an overview of what members can expect at group meetings. You can use the "Making It Happen" section on page 46 for brief descriptions of the meeting's elements. Also see "Things to Mention to Your Group about Weighing and Measuring" on page 57 to make sure your members know the reasons behind the weekly weigh-in.

   E. In a few words, review four-sided person concept.

3. Present the Wellness Spotlight (30 minutes).

   A. View the "Grocery Store Tour" and "In the Kitchen with the Dietitian" segments on the *Orientation and Food Plan* DVD. Assure members that they don't need to remember everything—these segments are introductory lessons for the Live It Plan. Suggest that member's read the *Member's Guide* for further details regarding the Live It Plan, which will also be covered in future meetings.

   B. View the "Understanding Your Live It Tracker" segment on the *Orientation and Food Plan* DVD and direct members to "Using Your Live It Tracker" (page 124 in the *Member's Guide*) for written instructions on how to complete it. Inform members that they will begin to use their Live It Trackers this first week. Reassure them that this is a learning experience and that progress, not perfection, is the goal. See page 64 for more infomation about the Live It Tracker.

   C. Introduce Live It Step 1: "*Learn* that Change Begins from the Inside Out." You will find "Step 1: *Learn*" on page 102 of the *Member's Guide*. Read the introduction aloud to your members or have a volunteer do so. Inform members that completion of Step 1 is part of their homework this week.

4. Assign homework and weekly challenge (2 to 3 minutes).
   Note: You may vary the method of presenting assignments for each week according to available time. You can assign them verbally, list them on a chalkboard or whiteboard, or type them out and give each member a copy.

   A. Assign the Live It Tracker Challenge: Challenge your members to fill out their Live It Tracker this week to the best of their ability. This may mean that they write down food choices but do not categorize them into food groups or specify amounts (cups, ounces, teaspoons). Assure them that their skills will develop with practice. Encourage them to begin using the Tracker to help them meet their short- and long-term goals.

   B. Remind members that two-week menu plans are included in the Bible study. Using these menu choices will help them adopt healthier eating habits and enable them to fill out the Live It Tracker with ease.

   C. Assign Bible study Week Two and the Scripture memory verse.

   D. Ask members to complete "Your Health Assessment" (page 112), "Nutrition for Life" (page 118) and "Step 1: *Learn*" (page 102) in the *Member's Guide*.

5. Have prayer time (10 to 12 minutes).

   A. Direct members to the Group Prayer Request Form in their Bible study. Use this form to record any special prayer requests given in each group meeting.

   B. Direct members to complete their Prayer Request Forms and place them in the container provided.

C. Direct each member to select randomly out of the container and pray for the selected person this week. Encourage members to contact their selected person once during the week by email or phone.

D. Close the meeting in group prayer.

AFTER THE MEETING

1. Complete a new Group Roster, incorporating any corrections, and photocopy for each member to hand out at next week's meeting.

2. After a few days, call members to see if they have questions concerning the Live It Tracker.

3. Check for accuracy on the Weigh-in/Measurements Chart.

4. Contact absentee members and arrange a time for them to view the "Grocery Store Tour," "In the Kitchen with the Dietitian" and "Understanding Your Live It Tracker" segments on the *Orientation and Food Plan* DVD.

5. Review the completed Member Surveys. Make note of those members who are willing to assist you or who have a special talent they would like to share with the group.

member weigh-in/ measurements

Some form of accountability in all four areas, including the physical aspect of a healthy weight, is important for a member's motivation and commitment levels. Unfortunately, too often in our society the scale has been misused and misrepresented as the *only* meaningful form of health assessment. This simply isn't true—there are many methods for keeping tabs on our physical health, such as blood lipid and blood glucose tolerance testing, Body Mass Index (BMI), fitness testing, and even a subjective assessment of sleep quality.

However, measuring body weight is one of the easiest, cheapest and most efficient methods for providing a general snapshot of one's health. Taking body circumference measurements is another easy and efficient tool, and one that often serves as a better barometer of health than the scale. These numbers should always be considered in conjunction with other health assessment information, but in the interest of time and resources, they are appropriate measures for your group to monitor during the session.

THINGS TO MENTION TO YOUR GROUP ABOUT WEIGHING AND MEASURING

1. *The scale doesn't just weigh fat.* It weighs muscle, bone, water, internal organs and all. When you lose "weight," that doesn't necessarily mean that you've lost fat. In fact, the scale has no way of telling you what you've lost (or gained).

2. If you are exercising and eating right, *don't be discouraged by a small gain on the scale.* Fluctuations are perfectly normal. Expect them to happen and take them in stride.

3. Exercise physiologists tell us that in order to store one pound of fat, you need to eat 3,500 calories more than your body is able to burn. But have you ever noticed that sometimes the scale shows you've gained 3 or 4 pounds overnight? For you to gain 4 pounds of fat in one day, you would have to consume a whopping 14,000 calories. This is not

likely—in fact, it's impossible. *So when the scale goes up 3 or 4 pounds overnight, rest easy . . . it's likely to be water, glycogen and the weight of your dinner.* Keep in mind that the 3,500-calorie rule also works in reverse. In order to lose one pound of fat, you must burn 3,500 calories more than you take in. Generally, it's only possible to lose 1 to 2 pounds of fat per week. When you follow a very low calorie diet that causes your weight to drop 10 pounds in 7 days, it's physically impossible for all of that to be fat. What you're really losing is water, glycogen and muscle.

4. *The best measurement tool of all may be your very own eyes.* How do you look? How do you feel? How do your clothes fit? Are your rings looser? Do your muscles feel firmer?

5. *Body measurements are often more discreet and take longer to appear than changes on the scale.* Take measurements at the beginning and end of your session (Week One and Week Twelve).

6. *A loss of inches is often a better barometer of healthy living,* especially inches lost around the waist/abdomen. Women should aim for a waist circumference of less than 35 inches, and men less than 40.

WEIGH-IN GUIDELINES

The majority of your class members will most likely choose to weigh in each week. Keep the following guidelines in mind:

1. Keep the Weigh-in/Measurements Chart concealed in a notebook or folder. Never leave it out where someone can see it.

2. Weigh members in private. If possible, place the scale in a separate room or in a private area of your classroom. Don't say the member's weight aloud; discreetly write the number on the Chart.

3. Encourage members to record their weekly weight, baseline and last-session measurements on the Personal Weight and Measurement Record located in their Bible Study.

4. Ask members to recite their memory verse as they are weighed.

5. Weigh members in an accurate and swift manner. Return the scale to zero before the next member is weighed.

6. Be sensitive and encouraging as members weigh. Do not show a reaction to the weight on the scale, but respond to the member.

7. When each member is finished weighing, remind them to turn in their Live It Tracker.

8. The Weigh-in/Measurements Chart also serves as an attendance record. Occasionally a member may not want to weigh in for various reasons. Always encourage him or her to view weighing in as an opportunity for a fresh start, but be sensitive and don't insist. Simply mark him or her present on the chart.

9. Weigh late arrivals after class. An exception is a lunchtime meeting, when members may want to weigh before they eat.

While weighing each week is the most common method of measuring weight loss, it is not always the best way for everyone. For example, members who have a history of anorexia nervosa or bulimia nervosa should be treated with sensitivity in this matter. Be sure to consult with these members privately and get their feedback—it may be counter-productive for them to weigh-in every week. Weighing backward, so they cannot see the scale, is one potential solution for reducing any anxiety or fear they may experience.

MEASUREMENTS GUIDELINES

1. Purchase several easy-to-read cloth or soft plastic tape measures.

2. Measure the member instead of letting them take their own measurements. The most accurate measurement comes from someone other than the member.

3. If you have time before your group meeting, train a few volunteer members so that this process goes more quickly.

4. When measuring, hold the tape measure firmly, but do not pull or squeeze too tightly. Make sure the person is standing with their weight evenly distributed, with legs shoulder-width apart, not tense or "sucking in," but relaxed.

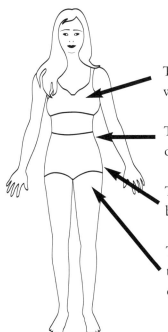

To measure chest/bust, wrap the tape measure around where chest/bust is widest.

To measure waist, wrap the tape measure around about one inch above the belly button.

To measure hips, wrap the tape measure around where buttocks are widest.

To measure thighs, wrap the tape measure around upper thigh and have the member place their weight on the opposite leg (that is, the leg being measured is relaxed).

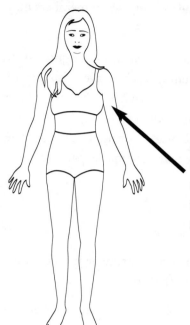

To measure arms, wrap the tape measure around the mid-upper portion of the person's arm, about halfway between the tip of their shoulder and the point of their elbow when at 90 degrees. Make sure that the person is relaxed and that their arm is hanging loosely by their side, palms facing thighs.

FREQUENTLY ASKED QUESTIONS

Q: *I have a member who has an aversion to the scale. Does he/she have to weigh in?*

A: People do better when they have some form of physical accountability. Weighing is the cheapest and most convenient way to monitor a person's progress toward their weight-loss goals. Nonetheless, if you have someone with a real aversion to the scale, suggest they weigh in at Weeks One, Six and Eleven. Or ask if they'd feel more comfortable weighing backward so they cannot see the scale. Remember to be sensitive if you encounter a member who is afraid to weigh in. Pray for the demolishing of this stronghold in their life and wait patiently as God does His work in them (see 2 Cor. 10:3-5).

Q: *How should I advise a member in my group who has a lot of weight to lose—more than 100 pounds?*

A: First, encourage them not to give up despite the long road ahead. We have testimonies on our website from people who have successfully lost more than 100 pounds in First Place 4 Health and kept it off for good! Share these stories with such members as inspiration. Second, refer them to page 118 in the *Member's Guide*, which explains calorie needs. It is very important that they choose a realistic and appropriate calorie level, not only to ensure that they can follow through, but for safety reasons too. Last, these individuals will likely lose more water weight at the beginning than others who have less to lose. After a few weeks, encourage them to mind the recommendation to lose no more than 2 pounds per week.

Q: *I have members who have lost weight and gained it back. How can I help them lose and maintain?*

A: National statistics tell us that 95 percent of people who lose weight gain it back. This is discouraging news, but it is a reality we will likely experience in First Place 4 Health from time to time. The only thing we can do is encourage members to begin again. As they learn how to give Christ first place in this area, He will help them lose weight and keep it off forever.

Sample Weigh-in/Measurements Chart

Weigh-in/Measurements Chart

Leader _____ Day _____ Time _____

Member Name	Weight Loss Goal	Week 1	Week 2	Week 3	Week 4	Week 5	Week 6	Week 7	Week 8	Week 9	Week 10	Week 11	Week 12

Beginning Measurements ~ Week 1: Chest _____ Waist _____ Hips _____ Thighs _____ Arms _____
Ending Measurements ~ Week 12: Chest _____ Waist _____ Hips _____ Thighs _____ Arms _____

Weekly Loss													
Session Loss Thus Far													

Beginning Measurements ~ Week 1: Chest _____ Waist _____ Hips _____ Thighs _____ Arms _____
Ending Measurements ~ Week 12: Chest _____ Waist _____ Hips _____ Thighs _____ Arms _____

Weekly Loss													
Session Loss Thus Far													

Beginning Measurements ~ Week 1: Chest _____ Waist _____ Hips _____ Thighs _____ Arms _____
Ending Measurements ~ Week 12: Chest _____ Waist _____ Hips _____ Thighs _____ Arms _____

Weekly Loss													
Session Loss Thus Far													

Beginning Measurements ~ Week 1: Chest _____ Waist _____ Hips _____ Thighs _____ Arms _____
Ending Measurements ~ Week 12: Chest _____ Waist _____ Hips _____ Thighs _____ Arms _____

Weekly Loss													
Session Loss Thus Far													

inside the member's kit

In your group's very first meeting (Week One), walk your members through the contents of their Member's Kits. (You may need to schedule 10 to 15 minutes before or after your regular meeting time to do this, as there is a lot to cover in Week One.) Make sure members understand how each component works with the others to help them bring balance and health to each facet of themselves—physical, mental, emotional and spiritual.

The First Place 4 Health Member's Kit includes the following elements:

- *First Place 4 Health Member's Guide*

- *First Place 4 Health* (by Carole Lewis with Marcus Brotherton)

- *Simple Ideas for Healthy Living*

- *Food on the Go Pocket Guide*

- *First Place 4 Health Prayer Journal*

- *Emotions and Eating* DVD

- *Why Should a Christian Be Physically Fit?* DVD

Descriptions of each of these products can be found on pages 18-19.

Make sure that each member also has a copy of the First Place 4 Health Bible study that has been selected for the current 12-week session. (A Bible study is not included in the Member's Kit because a new study is used for each session.) Let them know how the Bible study works: Members study a specific area of the Bible for an entire week and then answer questions to help them learn what the text means. Each week has five days of questions related to the Scriptures they are studying, then two days reserved for reflecting on what they have learned that week and on how to apply it. (Encourage them to read "Studying Scripture" in the *First Place 4 Health Member's Guide* for more information about using their Bible study.)

When your members understand how to use their materials individually, let them know what they can expect from each week's group meeting.

FREQUENTLY ASKED QUESTIONS

Q: *What is the best way to handle dropouts?*

A: On occasion, people join First Place 4 Health and later realize they cannot fulfill their commitment. Encourage them to continue, but if they decide to drop out, don't hesitate to ask them to consider joining again in the future. Through notes and/or phone calls, keep the door open for members to return at a later session.

the
live it tracker!

The Live It Tracker is a tool by which First Place 4 Health members can keep a record of their nutrition and physical activities as well as their spiritual disciplines. Completing their Tracker is an exercise in practicing mindfulness and is meant to assist them in their weight-loss or maintenance journey.

As a leader of First Place 4 Health, one of your most important roles is that of encourager. One of the main reasons we ask members to turn in their Trackers is so that they can receive constructive feedback and direction. Keep this in mind when you evaluate your members' Live It Trackers. Make sure your members understand that their Live It Tracker is a tool *for them* to monitor their progress. The more they see it as an activity designed to help them reach their goals and less one that must be "graded," the more likely they will be to utilize it and take it seriously.

1 Look first to see if the Tracker is complete. Did the member keep track of his or her food intake and physical and spiritual activities each day?

2 Next, consider the member's weekly goals. Are they realistic? Too difficult? Too easy? Before making suggestions or recommendations, compare several weeks' worth of Live It Trackers to help you assess these goals accurately. If a member consistently falls short of his or her physical activity goal, for instance, it may be that he or she needs to set a more reasonable goal for this area.

3 Look for obvious trouble spots. For example, if a member's Tracker alerts you that they are not eating enough or are eliminating an entire food group, bring this to his or her attention. Be on the lookout for evidence that he or she needs direction from you with regard to eating or exercise habits.

As previously noted, each First Place 4 Health Bible study contains 12 one-page Live It Trackers. Each single-page Tracker can be used by members to record information for each of the seven days in that week of the study. The following is a sample "expanded" single-day version (also available at www.firstplace4health.com).

Live It Tracker

Name: _____

Date: _____ Week #: _____ Calorie Range: _____

My week at a glance: ❑ Great ❑ So-so ❑ Not so great

My food goal for next week: _____

Activity Level: ❑ None ❑ < 30 min/day ❑ 30-60 min/day ❑ 60+ min/day

My activity goal for next week: _____

Scripture Memory Verse: _____

_____

RECOMMENDED DAILY AMOUNT OF FOOD FROM EACH GROUP:

Group	Daily Calories							
	1300-1400	1500-1600	1700-1800	1900-2000	2100-2200	2300-2400	2500-2600	2700-2800
Fruits	1.5-2 c.	1.5-2 c.	1.5-2 c.	2-2.5 c.	2- 2.5 c.	2.5- 3.5 c.	3.5- 4.5 c.	3.5- 4.5 c.
Vegetables	1.5-2 c.	2-2.5 c.	2.5-3 c.	2.5-3 c.	3- 3.5 c.	3.5- 4.5 c.	4.5- 5 c.	4.5- 5 c.
Grains	5 oz-eq.	5-6 oz-eq.	6-7 oz-eq.	6-7 oz-eq.	7- 8 oz-eq.	8-9 oz-eq.	9-10 oz-eq.	10-11 oz-eq.
Milk	2- 3 c.	3 c.	3 c.	3 c.	3 c.	3 c.	3 c.	3 c.
Meat & Beans	4 oz-eq.	5 oz-eq.	5- 5.5 oz-eq.	5.5- 6.5 oz-eq.	6.5- 7 oz-eq.	7 -7.5 oz-eq.	7- 7.5 oz-eq.	7.5- 8 oz-eq.
Healthy Oils	4 tsp.	5 tsp.	5 tsp.	6 tsp.	6 tsp.	7 tsp.	8 tsp.	8 tsp.

FOOD CHOICES

Breakfast: _____

_____

_____

_____

Lunch: _____

_____

_____

_____

Dinner: _____

_____

_____

_____

_____

Live It Tracker

4 first place
health
discover a new way to healthy living

Snacks:

_____
_____
_____
_____
_____

Group	Fruits	Vegetables	Grains
Goal Amount			
Estimate Your Total			
Increase ⇧ or Decrease⇩?			

Group	Meat & Beans	Milk	Oils
Goal Amount			
Estimate Your Total			
Increase ⇧ or Decrease⇩?			

PHYSICAL ACTIVITY

Description:

_____
_____
_____
_____
_____

Steps/Miles/Minutes: _____

SPIRITUAL ACTIVITY

Description:

_____
_____
_____
_____
_____
_____

Refrain from marking up your members' Trackers with unessential notes and instructions. Focus on the positive and—at most—three suggestions for improvement. As you learn how to give constructive and encouraging feedback, your members will realize how wonderful it is to have someone in their corner, cheering for them to make better choices each week!

FREQUENTLY ASKED QUESTIONS

Q: *I have a member who loves the spiritual aspect of class (Bible study, prayer support, Scripture memory), but just doesn't do the Live It Tracker! How should I handle this situation?*

A: Remember that First Place 4 Health is a four-sided program. God might want to work for a while on that person in an area other than the physical aspect of the program. Be patient and keep encouraging them to embrace the whole program, but know that God may simply have a few more lessons to teach the person before He moves on to other areas. The goal is to keep the person from dropping out before they find the success they originally came for. We like to say, "If you don't quit, you will succeed. Success is found in the process, not the program." Enjoy watching God work with each and every person in your group, and remember that His ways are higher than ours (see Isaiah 55:8-9)

meeting outlines

week two meeting outline

BEFORE THE MEETING

1. Review Live It Step 1, "*Learn* that Change Begins from the Inside Out," and familiarize yourself with Live It Step 2, "*Choose* to Set Yourself Up for Success," the "Quiet Time" segment of the *Orientation and Food Plan* DVD and the Quiet Time Challenge.

2. Memorize the Scripture memory verse and complete Week Two of the Bible study. Use the Leader Discussion Guide at the back of the Bible study to prepare a discussion.

3. Call members to ask if they have any questions about last week's lesson, specifically about filling out their Live It Tracker, completing their personal health assessment or determining a healthy calorie range.

4. Pray for group members.

5. Purchase some kind of reward/incentive to encourage members who complete their Live It Trackers and memorize the memory verse.

6. Make copies of the Group Roster for each member with corrected information.

7. Arrive early to set up the meeting room with chairs and tables.

   A. Set up the TV and DVD player and cue the DVD so that it is ready for viewing during the meeting.
   B. Place a Group Roster on each chair.
   C. Have extra pens or pencils, paper and Bibles available for those who may have forgotten them.
   D. Have nametags sitting out for members when they arrive.

THE MEETING

1. Complete arrival activities (15 minutes).

   A. Greet members.

   B. Privately weigh and/or measure each member and record weights and/or measurements on the Weigh-in/Measurements Chart. Listen to their Scripture memory verse recitations.

   C. Collect completed Live It Trackers.

2. Open the meeting (5 minutes).

   A. Open with prayer.

   B. Begin with one or both of the following icebreaker activities:

      1. Ask members to share what they hope to learn/accomplish during the next 11 weeks.
      2. Ask members to find a partner and find out a little more about the other person (hobbies, goals, random facts).

3. Present the Wellness Spotlight (10 minutes).

   A. Briefly review Live It Step 1 and ask a few members to share their answers to the three questions *Why are you overweight? Why do you want to lose weight?* and *If you've lost weight in the past, why did you gain it back?*

   B. Introduce Live It Step 2, "*Choose* to Set Yourself Up for Success." Read the introduction to "Step 2: *Choose*" (*Member's Guide*, page 104) aloud, or have a volunteer read it. Inform members that completion of Step 2 is part of their homework this week.

4. View the "Quiet Time" segment of the *Orientation and Food Plan* DVD (4 minutes). This segment is intended to inspire members to prepare and prioritize a consistent, daily quiet time with God. Conclude the viewing of this segment with encouragement and personal testimony regarding the importance of having personal time with God each day.

5. Lead Bible study discussion (25 minutes). From the Leader Discussion Guide in the back of the Bible study, pick two or three major ideas or application items to discuss regarding this week's study. (If you try to cover everything, you will likely run out of time and have only a superficial discussion.) Pose open-ended questions and encourage group interaction.

6. Assign homework and weekly challenge (2 to 3 minutes). Instruct members to complete the following assignments before the next meeting:

   A. Read "Step 2: *Choose*," *Member's Guide* page 104.

   B. Read "The Nutrition Top 10," *Member's Guide* page 109.

C. Read "The Fitness Top 10," *Member's Guide* page 180.

D. Complete Week Three of the Bible Study.

E. Memorize this week's Scripture memory verse.

F. Take the Quiet Time Challenge. Challenge members to find a special spot where they can set aside a special time each day this week for their quiet time. Encourage them to be creative and specific when planning their quiet times. If your members are already having a consistent quiet time, challenge them to "think outside the box" this week and try something new, such as accompanying their Scripture reading with a biblical commentary, listening to passages read aloud on CD, or doing something creative (painting, dancing, drawing) to worship God.

7. Have prayer time (10 minutes).

A. Direct members to the Group Prayer Request Form in their Bible study. Use this form to record any special prayer requests given in each group meeting.

B. Direct members to complete their Prayer Request Forms and place them in the container provided.

C. Direct each member to select randomly out of the container and pray for the selected person this week. Encourage members to contact their selected person once during the week by email or phone.

D. Close the meeting in group prayer.

AFTER THE MEETING

1. Evaluate members' Live It Trackers. Remember to be positive with any comments. (Refer to "The Live It Tracker" on page 64 for evaluation guidelines.)

2. Calculate weight loss for each member, and determine the group total for the week. Check for accuracy on the Weigh-in/Measurements Chart.

3. Contact absentee members by phone, email or a personal note, encouraging them to attend next week and giving them information about the homework and weekly challenge assignments.

week three meeting outline

BEFORE THE MEETING

1. Review Live It Step 2, "*Choose* to Set Yourself Up for Success," familiarize yourself with Live It Step 3, "*Use* the Tools Provided in the Live It Plan," view "The Nutrition Top 10"

segment of the *Orientation and Food Plan* DVD and familiarize yourself with the Nutrition Top 10 Challenge.

2. Memorize the Scripture memory verse and complete Week Three of the Bible study. Use the Leader Discussion Guide at the back of the Bible study to prepare a discussion.

3. Call members to ask if they have any questions about last week's lesson, specifically about the Nutrition and Fitness Top 10 lists, Live It Step 2 or how to have a quiet time.

4. Pray for group members.

5. Arrive early to set up the meeting room with chairs and tables.

    A. Set up the TV and DVD player and cue the DVD so that it is ready for viewing during the meeting.
    B. Have extra pens or pencils, paper and Bibles available for those who may have forgotten them.
    C. Have nametags sitting out for members when they arrive.

THE MEETING

1. Complete arrival activities (15 minutes).

    A. Greet members.
    B. Privately weigh and/or measure each member and record weights and/or measurements on the Weigh-in/Measurements Chart. Listen to their Scripture memory verse recitations.
    C. Collect completed Live It Trackers and return last week's evaluated Live It Trackers.
    D. Open the meeting in prayer.

2. Present the Wellness Spotlight (35 minutes).

    A. Briefly review Live It Step 2 and ask a few members to share their experience completing the three tasks: (1) *Clear out "toxic" foods from your immediate physical environment,* (2) *Make a list of food-free activities that you consider treats,* and (3) *Get support.*
    B. Introduce Live It Step 3, "*Use* the tools provided by the Live It Plan." Read the introduction to "Step 3: *Use*" (*Member's Guide,* page 108) aloud or have a volunteer read it. Inform members that completion of Step 3 is part of their homework this week.
    C. View "The Nutrition Top 10" segment of the *Orientation and Food Plan* DVD. Encourage your members to learn the Nutrition Top 10 and remind them that many of these behaviors are relatively simple to adopt—they just take practice and a conscientious effort to become second nature.

3. Lead Bible study discussion (25 minutes). From the Leader Discussion Guide in the back of the Bible study, pick two or three major ideas or application items to discuss

regarding this week's study. (If you try to cover everything, you will likely run out of time and have only a superficial discussion.) Pose open-ended questions and encourage group interaction.

4. Assign homework and weekly challenge (2 to 3 minutes). Instruct members to complete the following assignments before the next meeting:

    A. Read "Step 3: *Use*," *Member's Guide* page 108.
    B. Read and complete "The Benefits of Physical Activity," *Member's Guide* page 182.
    C. View *Why Should a Christian Be Physically Fit?* DVD.
    D. Complete Week Four of the Bible Study.
    E. Memorize this week's Scripture memory verse.
    F. Take the Nutrition Top 10 Challenge. Remind your members that the Nutrition Top 10 is a fundamental part of the Live It nutrition plan, and that mastery of the 10 behaviors listed will greatly increase their rate of successful weight loss and maintenance. Challenge your members to note on their Live It Tracker how many of the Nutrition Top 10 they achieve daily for one week. Achieving even one consistently each day is better than achieving none, but challenge them to adopt most of the, if not the entire, list of 10.

5. Have prayer time (10 minutes).

    A. Direct members to the Group Prayer Request Form in their Bible study. Use this form to record any special prayer requests given in each group meeting.
    B. Direct members to complete their Prayer Request Forms and place them in the container provided.
    C. Direct each member to select randomly out of the container and pray for the selected person this week. Encourage members to contact their selected person once during the week by email or phone.
    D. Close the meeting in group prayer.

AFTER THE MEETING

1. Evaluate members' Live It Trackers. Remember to be positive with any comments. (Refer to "The Live It Tracker" on page 64 for evaluation guidelines.)

2. Calculate weight loss for each member, and determine the group total for the week. Check for accuracy on the Weigh-in/Measurements Chart.

3. Contact absentee members by phone, email or a personal note, encouraging them to attend next week and giving them information about the homework and weekly challenge assignments.

week four meeting outline

BEFORE THE MEETING

1. Review Live It Step 3, "*Use* the Tools Provided by the Live It Plan," view "The Fitness Top 10" segment of the *Orientation and Food Plan* DVD, read through "Grocery Shopping Tips" (*Member's Guide*, page 176), and familiarize yourself with the Grocery Store and Fitness Challenges.

2. Memorize the Scripture memory verse and complete Week Four of the Bible study. Use the Leader Discussion Guide at the back of the Bible study to prepare a discussion.

3. Call members to ask if they have any questions about last week's lesson, specifically about Live It Step 3, "The Benefits of Physical Activity" and *Why Should a Christian Be Physically Fit?* DVD.

4. Pray for group members.

5. Arrive early to set up the meeting room with chairs and tables.
   A. Set up the TV and DVD player and cue the DVD so that it is ready for viewing during the meeting.
   B. Have extra pens or pencils, paper and Bibles available for those who may have forgotten them.
   C. Have nametags sitting out for members when they arrive.

THE MEETING

1. Complete arrival activities (15 minutes).
   A. Greet members.
   B. Privately weigh and/or measure each member and record weights and/or measurements on the Weigh-in/Measurements Chart. Listen to their Scripture memory verse recitations.
   C. Collect completed Live It Trackers and return last week's evaluated Live It Trackers.
   D. Open the meeting in prayer.

2. Present the Wellness Spotlight (20 minutes).
   A. Briefly review Live It Step 3 and ask for a few members to share their experience completing Step 3, specifically putting the Live It Nutrition plan into practice.
   B. View "The Fitness Top 10" segment on the *Orientation and Food Plan* DVD. The Fitness Top 10 is a list of practical tips to help members adopt a safe and effective

fitness lifestyle. For example, number 9 encourages consistency in their exercise activities as fundamental for members' success in developing and maintaining their personal exercise plan. Encourage your members to identify which of the Fitness Top 10 will be most helpful to them.

C. Introduce "Grocery Shopping Tips" (*Member's Guide* page 176). Encourage your members to jot down some of the tips discussed and bring them with them to the grocery store when they shop next. Putting into practice what we know is the basis for real behavior change, so explain how practical and important this week's wellness spotlight is for making real and lasting lifestyle change.

3. Lead Bible study discussion (25 minutes). From the Leader Discussion Guide in the back of the Bible study, pick two or three major ideas or application items to discuss regarding this week's study. (If you try to cover everything, you will likely run out of time and have only a superficial discussion.) Pose open-ended questions and encourage group interaction.

4. Assign homework and weekly challenge (2 to 3 minutes). Instruct members to complete the following assignments before the next meeting:

A. Read and complete "Starting a Basic Exercise Program," *Member's Guide* page 185.

B. Take the Grocery Store and Fitness Challenges. During their trip(s) to the grocery store this week, encourage your members to get better acquainted with sections they might not be used to frequenting, such as the produce section, whole-grain section of the bread aisle or the section of the meat department where lean and extra-lean cuts of meat are found. Also encourage them to try something new that they know is healthy but may have been intimidated to try in the past, such as an uncommon vegetable, fruit or high-fiber cereal. For the Fitness Challenge, encourage members to do *at least* 15 minutes of a physical activity of their choice six times this week.

C. Complete Week Five of the Bible Study.

D. Memorize this week's Scripture memory verse.

5. Have prayer time (10 minutes).

A. Direct members to the Group Prayer Request Form in their Bible study. Use this form to record any special prayer requests given in each group meeting.

B. Direct members to complete their Prayer Request Forms and place them in the container provided.

C. Direct each member to select randomly out of the container and pray for the selected person this week. Encourage members to contact their selected person once during the week by email or phone.

D. Close the meeting in group prayer.

AFTER THE MEETING

1. Evaluate members' Live It Trackers. Remember to be positive with any comments. (Refer to "The Live It Tracker" on page 64 for evaluation guidelines.)
2. Calculate weight loss for each member, and determine the group total for the week. Check for accuracy on the Weigh-in/Measurements Chart.
3. Contact absentee members by phone, email or a personal note, encouraging them to attend next week and giving them information about the homework and weekly challenge assignments.

week five meeting outline

BEFORE THE MEETING

1. Read "Understanding the Nutrition Facts Panel" (*Member's Guide* page 149), and review "The Benefits of Physical Activity" (*Member's Guide* page 182) and the Food Label Challenge.

2. Memorize the Scripture memory verse and complete Week Five of the Bible study. Use the Leader Discussion Guide at the back of the Bible study to prepare a discussion.

3. Call members to ask if they have any questions about last week's lesson, specifically about starting a basic exercise program and the Grocery Store and Fitness Challenges.

4. Pray for group members.

5. Arrive early to set up the meeting room with chairs and tables.
    A. Have extra pens or pencils, paper and Bibles available for those who may have forgotten them.
    B. Have nametags sitting out for members when they arrive.
    C. Print out sample food labels as visual aids for each member so that they can follow along as you present "Understanding the Nutrition Facts Panel."

THE MEETING

1. Complete arrival activities (15 minutes).
    A. Greet members.
    B. Privately weigh and/or measure each member and record weights and/or measurements on the Weigh-in/Measurements Chart. Listen to their Scripture memory verse recitations.

C. Collect completed Live It Trackers and return last week's evaluated Live It Trackers.

D. Open the meeting in prayer.

2. Present the Wellness Spotlight (25 minutes).

A. Ask for feedback regarding your members' experiences with the Grocery Store and Fitness Challenges.

B. Briefly review "The Benefits of Physical Activity" and ask for a few members to share what they wrote on page 184 of the *Member's Guide*.

C. Teach "Understanding the Nutrition Facts Panel" (*Member's Guide* page 149). Understanding how to read food labels is essential for selecting the best foods from a plethora of choices in today's supermarkets. Provide enough time for this lesson and take it piece by piece. Provide sample food labels for each group member to follow along with as you dissect the label line by line (serving size, total calories, grams of total fat, and so on) and explain each element's importance in making healthy choices.

3. Lead Bible study discussion (25 minutes). From the Leader Discussion Guide in the back of the Bible study, pick two or three major ideas or application items to discuss regarding this week's study. (If you try to cover everything, you will likely run out of time and have only a superficial discussion.) Pose open-ended questions and encourage group interaction.

4. Assign homework and weekly challenge (2 to 3 minutes). Instruct members to complete the following assignments before the next meeting:

A. Read "The Activity Pyramid" (*Member's Guide* page 190).

B. Take the Food Label Challenge. Understanding how to successfully read and interpret a food label is crucial in the search for the best and healthiest foods and beverages. Food labels exist not only on food packaging found in a grocery store, but most restaurants even offer a modified food label on their websites or in their establishments (usually in a binder or brochure) for all items sold. Challenge your members to read food labels this week before purchasing items, whether in the grocery store or in a restaurant. Encourage members to bring labels that they've read and/or obtained from restaurants to your meeting next week and explain what they learned. (For example, a member may bring in a nutrition facts panel for a cereal and explain that she chose the cereal because it provided more fiber than most others and contained little added sugar.)

C. Complete Week Six of the Bible Study.

D. Memorize this week's Scripture memory verse.

5. Have prayer time (10 minutes).

    A. Direct members to the Group Prayer Request Form in their Bible study. Use this form to record any special prayer requests given in each group meeting.

    B. Direct members to complete their Prayer Request Forms and place them in the container provided.

    C. Direct each member to select randomly out of the container and pray for the selected person this week. Encourage members to contact their selected person once during the week by email or phone.

    D. Close the meeting in group prayer.

AFTER THE MEETING

1. Evaluate members' Live It Trackers. Remember to be positive with any comments. (Refer to "The Live It Tracker" on page 64 for evaluation guidelines.)

2. Calculate weight loss for each member, and determine the group total for the week. Check for accuracy on the Weigh-in/Measurements Chart.

3. Contact absentee members by phone, email or a personal note, encouraging them to attend next week and giving them information about the homework and weekly challenge assignments.

week six meeting outline

BEFORE THE MEETING

1. Familiarize yourself with "Mapping Your Emotional History with Food" (*Member's Guide* page 90), "A Cure for Portion Distortion" (*Member's Guide* page 155) and the Emotional Challenge.

2. Memorize the Scripture memory verse and complete Week Six of the Bible study. Use the Leader Discussion Guide at the back of the Bible study to prepare a discussion.

3. Call members to ask if they have any questions about last week's lesson, specifically about "The Activity Pyramid" and the Food Label Challenge.

4. Pray for group members.

5. Arrive early to set up the meeting room with chairs and tables.

A. Have extra pens or pencils, paper and Bibles available for those who might have forgotten them.

B. Have nametags sitting out for members when they arrive.

THE MEETING

1. Complete arrival activities (15 minutes).

   A. Greet members.

   B. Privately weigh and/or measure each member and record weights and/or measurements on the Weigh-in/Measurements Chart. Listen to their Scripture memory verse recitations.

   C. Collect completed Live It Trackers and return last week's evaluated Live It Trackers.

   D. Open the meeting in prayer.

2. Present the Wellness Spotlight (20 minutes).

   A. Ask for feedback regarding your members' experiences with the Food Label Challenge.

   B. Teach "A Cure for Portion Distortion" (*Member's Guide* page 155). Many of your members will soon find out (if they haven't already) that they are simply eating too much. This wellness spotlight educates members regarding the widespread problem facing many Americans today: portion distortion. Use this time to focus on ways to escape the portion distortion traps abundant in our society, such as splitting food at restaurants, asking for healthy substitutions and separating appropriate portions into individual containers/baggies at home.

3. Lead Bible study discussion (25 minutes). From the Leader Discussion Guide in the back of the Bible study, pick two or three major ideas or application items to discuss regarding this week's study. (If you try to cover everything, you will likely run out of time and have only a superficial discussion.) Pose open-ended questions and encourage group interaction.

4. Assign homework and weekly challenge (2 to 3 minutes). Instruct members to complete the following assignments before the next meeting:

   A. View the "Emotional Mapping" section on the *Emotions and Eating* DVD. Cindy Schirle's message is extremely valuable for First Place 4 Health members. Encourage your members to watch the entire talk on DVD.

   B. Take the Emotional Mapping Challenge. After watching the DVD segment, encourage members to complete the emotional mapping activity found on page 90 of the *Member's Guide*.

   C. Complete Week Seven of the Bible Study.

   d. Memorize this week's Scripture memory verse.

5. Have prayer time (5 minutes).

   A. Direct members to the Group Prayer Request Form in their Bible study. Use this form to record any special prayer requests given in each group meeting.

   B. Direct members to complete their Prayer Request Forms and place them in the container provided.

   C. Direct each member to select randomly out of the container and pray for the selected person this week. Encourage members to contact their selected person once during the week by email or phone.

   D. Close the meeting in group prayer.

AFTER THE MEETING

1. Evaluate members' Live It Trackers. Remember to be positive with any comments. (Refer to "The Live It Tracker" on page 64 for evaluation guidelines.)

2. Calculate weight loss for each member, and determine the group total for the week. Check for accuracy on the Weigh-in/Measurements Chart.

3. Contact absentee members by phone, email or a personal note, encouraging them to attend next week and giving them information about the homework and weekly challenge assignments.

week seven meeting outline

BEFORE THE MEETING

1. Familiarize yourself with "Eating Healthy When Eating Out" (*Member's Guide* page 160), with "The FITT Formula for Exercise" (*Member's Guide* page 188) and with the Eating Out Challenge.

2. Memorize the Scripture memory verse and complete Week Seven of the Bible study. Use the Leader Discussion Guide at the back of the Bible study to prepare a discussion.

3. Call members to ask if they have any questions about last week's lesson, specifically about emotional mapping and the Emotional Challenge.

4. Pray for group members.

5. Arrive early to set up the meeting room with chairs and tables.

   A. Have extra pens or pencils, paper and Bibles available for those who might have forgotten them.

   B. Have nametags sitting out for members when they arrive.

THE MEETING

1. Complete arrival activities (15 minutes).
   A. Greet members.
   B. Privately weigh and/or measure each member and record weights and/or measurements on the Weigh-in/Measurements Chart. Listen to their Scripture memory verse recitations.
   C. Collect completed Live It Trackers and return last week's evaluated Live It Trackers.
   D. Open the meeting in prayer.

2. Present the Wellness Spotlight (25 minutes).
   A. Ask for feedback regarding your members' experiences with the Emotional Challenge.
   B. Teach "Eating Healthy When Eating Out" (*Member's Guide* page 160). One of the best things about this wellness spotlight is that it can be a very encouraging lesson for those who feel they have no control over what they are served when they eat out. On the contrary, they have much more power than they think and should exercise it without hesitation. We all have a right to eat healthy, and this can easily be achieved when eating out—we just have to ask the right questions! This wellness spotlight highlights many of those questions and other tactics for enjoying a meal out without a side of guilt!
   C. Discuss the four components of fitness and the FITT formula for exercise (*Member's Guide* page 188). Lead your class in understanding that in order to achieve and maintain as many health benefits as possible, cardio, strength and flexibility exercises all need to be a part of their personal exercise plan.

3. Lead Bible study discussion (20 minutes). From the Leader Discussion Guide in the back of the Bible study, pick two or three major ideas or application items to discuss regarding this week's study. (If you try to cover everything, you will likely run out of time and have only a superficial discussion.) Pose open-ended questions and encourage group interaction.

4. Assign homework and weekly challenge (2 to 3 minutes). Instruct members to complete the following assignments before the next meeting:
   A. Read and complete "My Prescription for Physical Fitness" (*Member's Guide* page 209).
   B. Take the Eating Out Challenge. Frequent eating out is a reality in America, but allowing it to sabotage your members' efforts can be prevented! Challenge them to adopt some of the tips and principles for healthy eating out discussed in "Eating Healthy When Eating Out," such as asking wait staff to prepare items more healthfully (e.g., dressing on the side, no butter on vegetables) or to split items before they arrive at the table. Have your members document the proactive deci-

sions they make when dining out during the coming week, and ask them to share their experiences at next week's meeting.

    C. Complete Week Eight of the Bible Study.

    D. Memorize this week's Scripture memory verse.

5. Have prayer time (10 minutes).

    A. Direct members to the Group Prayer Request Form in their Bible study. Use this form to record any special prayer requests given in each group meeting.

    B. Direct members to complete their Prayer Request Forms and place them in the container provided.

    C. Direct each member to select randomly out of the container and pray for the selected person this week. Encourage members to contact their selected person once during the week by email or phone.

    D. Close the meeting in group prayer.

AFTER THE MEETING

1. Evaluate members' Live It Trackers. Remember to be positive with any comments. (Refer to "The Live It Tracker" on page 64 for evaluation guidelines.)

2. Calculate weight loss for each member, and determine the group total for the week. Check for accuracy on the Weigh-in/Measurements Chart.

3. Contact absentee members by phone, email or a personal note, encouraging them to attend next week and giving them information about the homework and weekly challenge assignments.

week eight meeting outline

BEFORE THE MEETING

1. Familiarize yourself with "Cardiovascular Exercises" (*Member's Guide* page 193) and with the Pedometer/Walking/Aerobics Challenge.

2. Memorize the Scripture memory verse and complete Week Eight of the Bible study. Use the Leader Discussion Guide at the back of the Bible study to prepare a discussion.

3. Call members to ask if they have any questions about last week's lesson, specifically about "My Prescription for Physical Fitness" and the Eating Out Challenge.

4. Pray for group members.

5. Arrive early to set up the meeting room with chairs and tables.

    A. Have extra pens or pencils, paper and Bibles available for those who might have forgotten them.

    B. Have nametags sitting out for members when they arrive.

THE MEETING

1. Complete arrival activities (15 minutes).

    A. Greet members.

    B. Privately weigh and/or measure each member and record weights and/or measurements on the Weigh-in/Measurements Chart. Listen to their Scripture memory verse recitations.

    C. Collect completed Live It Trackers and return last week's evaluated Live It Trackers.

    D. Open the meeting in prayer.

2. Present the Wellness Spotlight (20 minutes).

    A. Ask for feedback regarding your members' experiences with the Eating Out Challenge.

    B. Teach "Cardiovascular Exercises" (*Member's Guide* page 193). Lead the class in understanding that the more active you are, the more calories you will burn.

3. Lead Bible study discussion (25 minutes). From the Leader Discussion Guide in the back of the Bible study, pick two or three major ideas or application items to discuss regarding this week's study. (If you try to cover everything, you will likely run out of time and have only a superficial discussion.) Pose open-ended questions and encourage group interaction.

4. Assign homework and weekly challenge (2 to 3 minutes). Instruct members to complete the following assignments before the next meeting:

    A. Take the Pedometer/Walking/Aerobics Challenge. Challenge members who use a pedometer to establish their base steps and add at least 100 steps each day of the week. Announce that there will be an award for the most creative ways to add steps (e.g., taking a walk as an extension of prayer time). For those not yet using a pedometer, challenge them to participate in an aerobic activity for at least 20 minutes (divided throughout the day or all together) *at least* three times in the coming week.

    B. Complete Week Nine of the Bible Study.

    C. Memorize this week's Scripture memory verse.

5. Have prayer time (10 minutes).

   A. Direct members to the Group Prayer Request Form in their Bible study. Use this form to record any special prayer requests given in each group meeting.

   B. Direct members to complete their Prayer Request Forms and place them in the container provided.

   C. Direct each member to select randomly out of the container and pray for the selected person this week. Encourage members to contact their selected person once during the week by email or phone.

   D. Close the meeting in group prayer.

AFTER THE MEETING

1. Evaluate members' Live It Trackers. Remember to be positive with any comments. (Refer to "The Live It Tracker" on page 64 for evaluation guidelines.)

2. Calculate weight loss for each member, and determine the group total for the week. Check for accuracy on the Weigh-in/Measurements Chart.

3. Contact absentee members by phone, email or a personal note, encouraging them to attend next week and giving them information about the homework and weekly challenge assignments.

week nine meeting outline

BEFORE THE MEETING

1. Familiarize yourself with "Strength Training" (*Member's Guide* page 201) and with the Strength Training Challenge.

2. Plan to give away a prize for the member with the most creative method for adding 100 steps per day for the Pedometer/Walking/Aerobics Challenge.

3. Memorize the Scripture memory verse and complete Week Nine of the Bible study. Use the Leader Discussion Guide at the back of the Bible study to prepare a discussion.

4. Call members to ask if they have any questions about last week's lesson, specifically about the Pedometer/Walking/Aerobics Challenge.

5. Pray for group members.

6. Arrive early to set up the meeting room with chairs and tables.

   A. Have extra pens or pencils, paper and Bibles available for those who might have forgotten them.

   B. Have nametags sitting out for members when they arrive.

THE MEETING

1. Complete arrival activities (15 minutes).

   A. Greet members.

   B. Privately weigh and/or measure each member and record weights and/or measurements on the Weigh-in/Measurements Chart. Listen to their Scripture memory verse recitations.

   C. Collect completed Live It Trackers and return last week's evaluated Live It Trackers.

   D. Open the meeting in prayer.

2. Present the Wellness Spotlight (20 minutes).

   A. Ask for feedback regarding your members' experiences with the Pedometer/Walking/Aerobics Challenge. Ask the members to vote for the most creative way a member found to add 100 steps per day, and give a prize to the winner.

   B. Teach "Strength Training" (*Member's Guide* page 201). Communicate to your class that strong muscles allow you to participate in more activities with ease and enjoyment, along with the added benefit of burning calories and building muscles.

3. Lead Bible study discussion (25 minutes). From the Leader Discussion Guide in the back of the Bible study, pick two or three major ideas or application items to discuss regarding this week's study. (If you try to cover everything, you will likely run out of time and have only a superficial discussion.) Pose open-ended questions and encourage group interaction.

4. Assign homework and weekly challenge (2 to 3 minutes). Instruct members to complete the following assignments before the next meeting:

   A. Take the Strength Training Challenge. Challenge your members to begin a strength training routine if they do not have one already. They can use free weights or machines at a gym, or purchase their own free weights or an inexpensive resistance band. Two sets of 10 repetitions with a light (but challenging) weight is a great start. Members who have already started a strength training routine are encouraged to exercise a new muscle group this week.

   B. Complete Week Ten of the Bible Study.

   C. Memorize this week's Scripture memory verse.

5. Have prayer time (10 minutes).

   A. Direct members to the Group Prayer Request Form in their Bible study. Use this form to record any special prayer requests given in each group meeting.

   B. Direct members to complete their Prayer Request Forms and place them in the container provided.

   C. Direct each member to select randomly out of the container and pray for the selected person this week. Encourage members to contact their selected person once during the week by email or phone.

   D. Close the meeting in group prayer.

AFTER THE MEETING

1. Evaluate members' Live It Trackers. Remember to be positive with any comments. (Refer to "The Live It Tracker" on page 64 for evaluation guidelines.)

2. Calculate weight loss for each member, and determine the group total for the week. Check for accuracy on the Weigh-in/Measurements Chart.

3. Contact absentee members by phone, email or a personal note, encouraging them to attend next week and giving them information about the homework and weekly challenge assignments.

week ten meeting outline

BEFORE THE MEETING

1. Familiarize yourself with "Flexibility and Balance Training" (*Member's Guide* page 205) and with the Flexibility and Balance Training Challenge.

2. Memorize the Scripture memory verse and complete Week Ten of the Bible study. Use the Leader Discussion Guide at the back of the Bible study to prepare a discussion.

3. Call members to ask if they have any questions about last week's lesson, specifically about the Strength Training Challenge.

4. Pray for group members.

5. Arrive early to set up the meeting room with chairs and tables.

   A. Have extra pens or pencils, paper and Bibles available for those who might have forgotten them.

   B. Have nametags sitting out for members when they arrive.

THE MEETING

1. Complete arrival activities (15 minutes).

   A. Greet members.

   B. Privately weigh and/or measure each member and record weights and/or measurements on the Weigh-in/Measurements Chart. Listen to their Scripture memory verse recitations.

   C. Collect completed Live It Trackers and return last week's evaluated Live It Trackers.

   D. Open the meeting in prayer.

2. Present the Wellness Spotlight (20 minutes).

   A. Ask for feedback regarding your members' experiences with the Strength Training Challenge.

   B. Teach "Flexibility and Balance Training" (*Member's Guide* page 205). Lead the group in understanding that flexibility exercises reduce pain and stiffness from their cardio workouts, prevent injuries and relieve the stress of everyday living.

3. Lead Bible study discussion (25 minutes). From the Leader Discussion Guide in the back of the Bible study, pick two or three major ideas or application items to discuss regarding this week's study. (If you try to cover everything, you will likely run out of time and have only a superficial discussion.) Pose open-ended questions and encourage group interaction.

4. Assign homework and weekly challenge (2 to 3 minutes). Instruct members to complete the following assignments before the next meeting:

   A. Take the Flexibility and Balance Training Challenge. Practice five minutes or more of stretching exercises while enjoying a television program. Also, practice getting up from a sitting position on the floor during every commercial break to improve balance.

   B. Complete Week Eleven of the Bible Study.

   C. Memorize this week's Scripture memory verse.

5. Have prayer time (10 minutes).

   A. Direct members to the Group Prayer Request Form in their Bible study. Use this form to record any special prayer requests given in each group meeting.

   B. Direct members to complete their Prayer Request Forms and place them in the container provided.

   C. Direct each member to select randomly out of the container and pray for the selected person this week. Encourage members to contact their selected person once during the week by email or phone.

   D. Close the meeting in group prayer.

AFTER THE MEETING

1. Evaluate members' Live It Trackers. Remember to be positive with any comments. (Refer to "The Live It Tracker" on page 64 for evaluation guidelines.)
2. Calculate weight loss for each member, and determine the group total for the week. Check for accuracy on the Weigh-in/Measurements Chart.
3. Contact absentee members by phone, email or a personal note, encouraging them to attend next week and giving them information about the homework and weekly challenge assignments.

week eleven meeting outline

BEFORE THE MEETING

1. Familiarize yourself with "Modifying Recipes" (*Member's Guide* page 165) and with the Extreme Recipe Makeover Challenge.

2. Memorize the Scripture memory verse and complete Week Eleven of the Bible study. Use the Leader Discussion Guide at the back of the Bible study to prepare a discussion.

3. Call members to ask if they have any questions about last week's lesson, specifically about the Flexibility and Balance Training Challenge.

4. Pray for group members.

5. Arrive early to set up the meeting room with chairs and tables.
   A. Have extra pens or pencils, paper and Bibles available for those who might have forgotten them.
   B. Have nametags sitting out for members when they arrive.

THE MEETING

1. Complete arrival activities (15 minutes).
   A. Greet members.
   B. Privately weigh and/or measure each member and record weights and/or measurements on the Weigh-in/Measurements Chart. Listen to their Scripture memory verse recitations.
   C. Collect completed Live It Trackers and return last week's evaluated Live It Trackers.
   D. Open the meeting in prayer.

2. Present the Wellness Spotlight (20 minutes).

    A. Ask for feedback regarding your members' experiences with the Flexibility and Balance Training Challenge.

    B. Teach "Modifying Recipes" (*Member's Guide* page 165). Lead the group in discovering how to improve the nutritional quality of recipes without having to sacrifice taste! Review the sample recipe makeovers provided in the *Member's Guide* and discuss what changes were made and the degree of their impact, nutritionally. Encourage your members to see cooking healthfully as an opportunity to make favorite family recipes even better!

3. Lead Bible study discussion (25 minutes). From the Leader Discussion Guide in the back of the Bible study, pick two or three major ideas or application items to discuss regarding this week's study. (If you try to cover everything, you will likely run out of time and have only a superficial discussion.) Pose open-ended questions and encourage group interaction.

4. Assign homework and weekly challenge (2 to 3 minutes). Instruct members to complete the following assignments before the next meeting:

    A. Take the Extreme Recipe Makeover Challenge. Remind your members that they don't have to discontinue making their favorite foods—they simply need to tweak them a bit so that they're healthy *and* delicious! Challenge your members to use the tips given in "Modifying Recipes" to shift their favorite recipes from the "guilty" category to "guilt-*free*"! Encourage members to bring their "before" and "after" recipes to class the following week to share with the group for the Victory Celebration!

    B. Complete Week Twelve of the Bible study.

5. Have prayer time (10 minutes).

    A. Direct members to the Group Prayer Request Form in their Bible study. Use this form to record any special prayer requests given in each group meeting.

    B. Direct members to complete their Prayer Request Forms and place them in the container provided.

    C. Direct each member to select randomly out of the container and pray for the selected person this week. Encourage members to contact their selected person once during the week by email or phone.

    D. Close the meeting in group prayer.

AFTER THE MEETING

1. Evaluate members' Live It Trackers. Remember to be positive with any comments. (Refer to "The Live It Tracker" on page 64 for evaluation guidelines.)

2. Calculate weight loss for each member, and determine the group total for the week. Check for accuracy on the Weigh-in/Measurements Chart.

3. Contact absentee members by phone, email or a personal note, encouraging them to attend next week and giving them information about the weekly challenge. Make sure to invite them to next week's Victory Celebration!

leading a first place 4 health
Bible study discussion

A Leader Discussion Guide is located in each First Place 4 Health Bible study. You will find many ideas for leading your group in a discussion about what they are learning in their personal study time. Below are some ideas to vary the ways you lead the discussion.

- Select just two or three of the ideas that appeal to you from the Leader Discussion Guide. There isn't enough time during the meeting to do all of them.

- Ask five people in your group to each talk about one day of the study. Do this a week ahead so that they have time to prepare.

- Break up into groups of two or three and ask each group to talk about one day of the study. After 5 minutes or so, have the larger group come back together and ask each small group to report what they liked best about their group's day.

- If someone checked on their Member Survey that they are willing to lead a Bible study discussion, ask them to lead one week. This develops potential leaders.

- Keep one member from dominating the discussion by saying something like, "That's a great idea. Thanks for sharing. Let's move on so that we have time to hear from everyone." Set up guidelines in the first meeting about respecting everyone's time. Remind members to keep their answers to one or two sentences. Communicate with members the importance of allowing everyone the opportunity to share in discussions. You may need to discuss the importance of this group dynamic one-on-one with people who consistently dominate discussions. People who monopolize meetings are usually crying out for attention. Try to give them additional attention outside of the group's meetings to reduce their need to monopolize as much.

- If one member asks a question that no one has the answer to, ask for a volunteer to research the answer and report back next week.

- Buy a rubber stamp that says "Great Job" or "Way to go!" at a teacher supply store. Stamp each member's Bible study when they come into the meeting. You might also put a sticker on it. This is "inspecting what we expect" and provides incentive for members to do their Bible study.

FREQUENTLY ASKED QUESTIONS

Q: *What if I have a shy person who does not want to participate in discussion?*

A: Be sensitive to people in your group who are shy and may feel embarrassed if called on to pray or speak during the meeting. Look for other ways to include them in the group. *Tip: Small-group or paired activities might help them feel safe and secure.*

creative meeting ideas

The following are some ideas for getting conversations started in your group meeting or activities that group members can do to help them think about their weight loss goals and the four core components of First Place 4 Health.

ICE BREAKERS

These are perfect if your members don't know each other well.

- Ask members to tell the group something that no one knows about them.
- Break up into groups of two and interview each other. After five minutes the two introduce each other, sharing the information they learned.
- Pick an animal whose name begins with your first initial (Julie/Jaguar, Carole/ Cat, Lisa/Leopard) and tell the group why the two of you are alike.
- Tell the group your favorite travel destination and why.

FOOD BANK FOOD RAISER

Ask each member to bring an amount of nonperishable packaged or canned food to the Victory Celebration equal to the amount of weight he or she has lost. Members are often amazed at the difficulty of carrying that amount of weight! Donate the food to a local food pantry.

FOOD CRITICS CORNER

Have each member find and research one restaurant in your area—you might want to assign them one. Have them evaluate the menu to see if it can be considered a "First Place 4 Health" restaurant. Examples could be 1 star = poor, 2 stars = fair, 3 stars = good, 4 stars = excellent and 5 stars = superior. Have members explain how they came to their evaluations.

POUND-O-FAT

Buy a pound of fat from your local butcher and put it in a clear plastic bag. Pass it around to let everyone see the significance of losing even one pound. Another idea is to hand out $1/4$ to $1/2$ pounds of fat in re-sealable bags for members to take home. This reminds members that even $1/4$ of a pound is significant.

BOOK FAIR

Ask members to bring a recipe book or any other book that has helped them while being in First Place 4 Health. Have each person briefly share how the book has helped them with the program. Books should be motivational and pertaining to one or more of the four areas of First Place: spiritual, emotional, physical or mental.

MEASURING MISHAPS

Bring a food scale and measuring cups and spoons to the meeting along with several foods that are often measured incorrectly, such as baked potatoes, meat, cheese, butter, mayonnaise, and the like. Let members estimate how many cups or ounces the food is without measuring it. Then measure the food to find the true measurement. This will encourage members to learn appropriate portion sizes.

THE HUMAN YO-YO

Provide a balloon for each member. Ask members to blow up balloons and let the air out several times. Call to their attention how much easier the balloon was to blow up each time, and how much larger it got each time. Compare this to the weight cycling, or yo-yo syndrome, of gaining and losing and gaining and losing. Suggest that members keep the balloons as reminders.

THE HARVEST

In a spring session, bring a package of fast-growing seeds, a package of soil and medium-sized paper cups to class. Set up a table where group members can plant their seeds in the paper cups. If necessary, provide directions for planting (see seed package). Begin the meeting by asking members what is necessary for the growth of this plant. Use the analogy that our spiritual lives are dependent on necessary components as well. Have the group use a concordance to do a word study on the words "grow," "growth" or "growing" in the Bible. Challenge members to nurture their plants and bring them to the Victory Celebration.

DINING-OUT FIELD TRIP

Meet at a restaurant instead of the usual meeting place. Discuss "Eating Healthy When Eating Out" in the *Member's Guide* (page 160) as you look over the menu and during the meal. Bring a scale, measuring cups and spoons for added fun!

SUPERMARKET SAVVY

Many grocery chains have people who give healthy-heart shopping tours. This is a wonderful field trip, if available in your area. If such a tour is not available, you can have a meeting that focuses on grocery planning and reading labels. Bring the grocery list provided in the *Member's Guide* or create a grocery list based on a few meals from the menu plans found in the back of your selected First Place 4 Health Bible study.

EXERCISE COMMITMENT

Invite a fitness professional such as an aerobic instructor or personal trainer to a group meeting and let him or her do the talking. You might even try meeting at the gym to turn the group into an aerobics class. Instruct members to wear appropriate exercise clothing.

PROFESSIONAL IMAGE CLASS

Call around to boutique-type apparel stores and ask if they have someone who can talk about fashion. Ask if they have any special knowledge about helping people look their best while reaching their goal weight. A makeover is always fun (even for men!). See if there is someone available who can do hair and makeup as well. You might want to choose one person in your class for a makeover. Be sure to take "before" and "after" pictures!

OUT WITH THE OLD, IN WITH THE RECYCLED!

After a group meeting, have a clothes swap. Many groups like to trade clothes as they lose weight. In this way, members can have a few new clothes as they work toward their goals.

SALAD LUNCHEON OR DINNER

This is a great way to celebrate success midway through a session. Everyone brings two cups of salad items and something to drink. Assign these items the week before. The leader could provide bowls, napkins and forks. Combine all the salad ingredients and serve 15 minutes before the meeting starts.

BAKED POTATO SUPPER

Another great way to celebrate is with a potato supper. Have each member sign up to bring a healthy potato topping. You provide the baked potatoes.

HALF-TIME PARTY

Midway through the session is a time when members' enthusiasm might start to falter. Week Six or Seven is a great time to bolster their confidence again. Choose a theme based on the season. You might want to share a meal or healthy dessert at the party. Give awards as you would at your Victory Celebration, but make them half-time specific, such as "Perfect Attendance," "Halfway to Goal" or "Recited Half the Memory Verses."

CLASS PRAYER TIME

If your time is short, ask members to write one-word prayer requests on their prayer request forms. These might be words like "exercise," "Tracker," "husband" or "daughter."

meeting outline

BEFORE THE MEETING

1. Familiarize yourself with the Maintenance Challenge.

2. Call members to ask if they have any questions about last week's lesson, specifically about modifying recipes and the Extreme Recipe Makeover Challenge. If they were assigned any duties, such as decorating or preparing a skit, for the Victory Celebration, remind them of the details.

3. Finalize plans for the Victory Celebration. For creative ideas, see page 98.

4. Pray for group members.

5. Arrive early to set up the meeting room. Have nametags sitting out for members when they arrive, and extras for visitors.

THE MEETING

1. Complete arrival activities (15 minutes).

    A. Greet members.
    B. Privately weigh and/or measure each member and record weights and/or measurements on the Weigh-in/Measurements Chart.
    C. Collect completed Live It Trackers and return last week's evaluated Live It Trackers.
    D. Open the meeting in prayer.

2. Present the Wellness Spotlight (30 minutes).

    A. Ask for feedback regarding your members' experiences with the Extreme Recipe Makeover Challenge. If any members brought samples of their "madeover" recipes, have them explain what modifications they made and how the dish turned out. Pass around small samples.

B. Give each of your members an opportunity to share a brief testimony about their experience with this 12-week session. See the Leader Discussion Guide in this session's Bible study for detailed instructions.

3. Assign the Maintenance Challenge (2 to 3 minutes). This challenge is the most important one thus far! Challenge your members to maintain their current weight or continue to lose more until the following session begins. (This is especially important if there are several weeks between sessions.) In order for them to succeed in this challenge, they must continue engaging in practical and meaningful healthy lifestyle activities (i.e., keeping a food record, exercising, splitting meals at restaurants). Encourage your members to make a list of the behaviors they plan to continue during the hiatus from First Place 4 Health meetings. Challenge them to share this list with an accountability partner who will stay in touch during the break.

4. Celebrate! It's party time! For creative ideas about throwing a Victory Celebration, see page 98.

5. Have prayer time (10 minutes).
   A. Give an opportunity for members to say a sentence or two of praise about what they are most thankful for about the last 12 weeks.
   B. Close the meeting in group prayer.

AFTER THE MEETING

1. Evaluate members' Live It Trackers. Remember to be positive with any comments. (Refer to "The Live It Tracker" on page 64 for evaluation guidelines.) Return members' Live It Trackers by mail with an encouraging note. Consider including the group's total weight loss over the past session.

2. Calculate weight loss for each member, and determine the group total for the week, as well as the entire session. Check for accuracy on the Weigh-in/Measurements Chart.

planning a victory celebration

A Victory Celebration is held at the end of each 12-week session. The following suggestions are provided to help get you started—but don't let these ideas limit your own creativity.

VICTORY DINNER OR LUNCHEON

Food may be catered, prepared in your church kitchen or provided by members. If you have First Place 4 Health funds available, you may want to provide the drinks and paper goods.

DECORATIONS

Ask for volunteers to make decorations and do the decorating.

You might want to decorate with a First Place 4 Health theme. For example, use First Place 4 Health mugs as vases, fill them with fresh flowers and give as rewards for leaders, assistants or group members.

If you took "Before" pictures, take "After" pictures. Buy an inexpensive double frame and use the pictures as table decorations. After the celebration, give the pictures to each member.

Tape measures make fun napkin rings: Cut a tape measure at 6-inch intervals and glue the ends together to make rings.

Another idea is to decorate with a holiday theme, depending on the time of year.

STYLE SHOW

Call members who have had a noticeable weight loss. Ask them to model something they wore before they lost weight. During the "style show," the narrator reads the models' testimony about what First Place 4 Health has meant to them. After models change into properly fitting clothes, they model again as the narrator shares how much weight/inches they have lost.

SPECIAL SPEAKER

Invite a speaker who will present an inspirational, educational or motivational message. The message could relate to any of the four areas of personal development covered in First Place 4 Health. *Caution:* It is a good idea to use speakers you have heard before.

SKITS

Present a skit. Ask volunteers from your class to develop and perform a skit on behavior modification, eating out or spiritual growth.

AWARDS TIME

Recognize each member's accomplishments. Present awards such as "Perfect Attendance," "Recited All 10 Memory Verses," "Most Consistent Member," "Exercise Award," "Live It Expert," "Prayer Warrior," "Reached Goal Weight," "Turned In Live It Tracker Each Week" or any other creative award. Be sure to give an award to every member. Consider special accomplishments, such as a diabetic who was faithful to a program to control blood sugar or a member who lowered his or her cholesterol. Successes in all areas should be recognized. The greatest victory of all is if a member accepted Jesus during the session. This would certainly constitute a very special recognition. Be sensitive to those members who are shy. Recognition should be done with respect for the individual's feelings. A sample First Place 4 Health award certificate is on page 101, which can be downloaded at www.firstplace4health.com.

TESTIMONY TIME

Invite members to give testimony about the changes God has helped them to make through First Place 4 Health. Plan these testimonies before the Victory Celebration. Give volunteers a five-minute time limit for their testimonies.

MUSIC

Ask someone in your group to provide special music.

BE CREATIVE

Be on the lookout for different options for your Victory Celebration. Network with other First Place 4 Health leaders in your area to gather ideas, or visit www.firstplace4health.com to connect with national and international leaders. Consider collaborating with other First Place 4 Health groups in your area for a "Victory Rally" to multiply the ministry and get the word out about First Place 4 Health.

VISITORS

Victory Celebrations are a great time for members to celebrate with their family and friends, or to bring guests who may be interested in joining First Place 4 Health.

Sample Award Certificate

first place
4health
discover a new way to healthy living

Presented to

for

Therefore, since we are surrounded by such a great cloud of witnesses,
let us throw off everything that hinders and the sin that so easily entangles,
and let us run with perseverance the race marked out for us.

Hebrews 12:1

Leading a First Place 4 Health Group Again

session outline

GO DEEPER

In order to prevent monotony and boredom in future classes, and to keep your class moving toward their wellness goals, we have provided you with a flexible teaching outline for subsequent 12-week sessions of First Place 4 Health. Certain learning activities should be repeated, as mastery of them is crucial to success in the program. These activities include explaining the Live It Tracker, Emotional Mapping and discussing Steps 1, 2 and 3 of the Live It Plan.

However, we have given you, the leader, some freedom with regard to how you execute your group meetings in weeks following the review of those activities. We understand that if you are teaching a group for the second, third or even tenth time, you know your group on a deeper level than we ever can and are aware of specific learning needs and desires of those faithful members. Therefore, with the necessary tools you will find throughout this guide to prepare and lead future sessions of First Place 4 Health, we encourage you to use your God-given abilities to tailor your meetings according to your group's needs, personality and dynamic.

You will find a "Weekly Lesson Plan" form on page 109 as well as a "Weekly Lesson Plan Master Outline" on page 110. You can use these to help you prepare for your meetings. Each of these resources is also available for download at www.firstplace4health.com.

Use *Simple Ideas for Healthy Living* and the *Member's Guide* as material for your wellness spotlights. Choose a topic that you believe is needed in your group and present a chapter that addresses that subject.

In the following pages, you will find a recommended list of various weekly challenges and homework activities to assign to your group. Instead of repeating the same challenges session after session, we encourage you to alternate those from the list that you think would be helpful or use them as a launching pad for your own creative ideas!

WEEK	LESSON PLAN	CHALLENGE AND HOMEWORK
One	1. Greet and weigh/measure members (15 minutes). 2. Review "The Four-Sided Person" (5 minutes). 3. View "Grocery Store Tour" and "In the Kitchen with the Dietitian" segments on the Orientation and Food Plan DVD (25 minutes). 4. View the "Using Your Live It Tracker" segment on the *Orientation and Food Plan* DVD (3 minutes). 5. Review Live It Step 1: "*Learn* that Change Begins from the Inside Out" (*Member's Guide* page 102, 2 minutes). 6. Assign homework (2-3 minutes). 7. Prayer (10 minutes).	1. Read "Step 1: *Learn*," *Member's Guide* page 102. 2. Complete "Your Health Assessment," *Member's Guide* page 112. 3. Complete "Nutrition for Life" to determine a calorie range, *Member's Guide* page 118. 4. Take the Live It Tracker Challenge. 5. Complete Week Two of the Bible study. 6. Memorize this week's Scripture memory verse.
Two	1. Greet and weigh members (15 minutes). 2. Review and discuss Live It Step 1 (5 minutes). 3. Review Live It Step 2: "*Choose* to Set Yourself Up for Success" (*Member's Guide* page 104, 5 minutes). 4. View the "Quiet Time" segment on the *Orientation and Food Plan* DVD (4 minutes). 5. Lead Bible study discussion (25 minutes). 6. Assign homework (2-3 minutes). 7. Prayer (10 minutes).	1. Read "Step 2: *Choose*," *Member's Guide* page 104. 2. Read "The Nutrition Top 10," *Member's Guide* page 109. 3. Read "The Fitness Top 10," *Member's Guide* page 180. 4. Take the Quiet Time Challenge. 5. Complete Week Three of the Bible study. 6. Memorize this week's Scripture memory verse.
Three	1. Greet and weigh members (15 minutes). 2. Review and discuss Live It Step 2 (5 minutes). 3. Review Live It Step 3, "*Use* the Tools Provided in the Live It Plan" (*Member's Guide* page 108, 5 minutes). 4. View "The Nutrition Top 10" segment on the *Orientation and Food Plan* DVD (17 minutes). 5. Lead Bible study discussion (25 minutes). 6. Assign homework (2-3 minutes). 7. Prayer (5 minutes).	1. Read "Step 3: *Use*," *Member's Guide* page 108. 2. Read and complete "The Benefits of Physical Activity," *Member's Guide* page 182. 3. View the *Why Should a Christian Be Physically Fit?* DVD. 4. Take the Nutrition Top 10 Challenge. 5. Complete Week Four of the Bible study. 6. Memorize this week's Scripture memory verse.
Four	1. Greet and weigh members (15 minutes). 2. Review and discuss Live It Step 3 (5 minutes). 3. View the "Fitness Top 10" segment on the *Orientation and Food Plan* DVD (6 minutes). 4. Review "Grocery Shopping Tips" (*Member's Guide* page 176, 5 minutes). 5. Lead Bible study discussion (25 minutes). 6. Assign homework (2-3 minutes). 7. Prayer (5 minutes).	1. Read "Starting a Basic Exercise Program," *Member's Guide* page 185. 2. Take the Grocery Store Challenge. 3. Take the Fitness Challenge. 4. Complete Week Five of the Bible study. 5. Memorize this week's Scripture memory verse.

WEEK	LESSON PLAN	CHALLENGE AND HOMEWORK
Five	1. Greet and weigh members (15 minutes). 2. Discuss the Grocery Store and Fitness Challenges (5 minutes). 3. Review and discuss "The Benefits of Physical Activity" exercise from Week Three (5 minutes). 4. Present a wellness spotlight of your own choosing (15 minutes). 5. Lead Bible study discussion (25 minutes). 6. Assign homework (2-3 minutes). 7. Prayer (5 minutes).	1. Read and complete "The Activity Pyramid," *Member's Guide* page 190. 2. Take the spiritual challenge chosen by the group leader. 3. Complete Week Six of the Bible study. 4. Memorize this week's Scripture memory verse.
Six	1. Greet and weigh members (15 minutes). 2. Discuss last week's challenge (5 minutes). 3. Present a wellness spotlight of your choosing (15 minutes). 4. Lead Bible study discussion (25 minutes). 5. Review "Mapping Your Emotional History with Food" (*Member's Guide* page 90, 5 minutes). 6. Assign homework (2-3 minutes). 7. Prayer (5 minutes).	1. View "Emotional Mapping" on the *Emotions and Eating* DVD (all three segments). 2. Take the emotional challenge chosen by the group leader. 3. Complete Week Seven of the Bible study. 4. Memorize this week's Scripture memory verse.
Seven	1. Greet and weigh members (15 minutes). 2. Discuss last week's challenge (5 minutes). 3. Present a wellness spotlight of your choosing (20 minutes). 5. Lead Bible study discussion (25 minutes). 6. Assign homework (2-3 minutes). 7. Prayer (5 minutes).	1. Review and complete "My Prescription for Personal Fitness," *Member's Guide* page 209. 2. Take the mental challenge chosen by the group leader. 3. Complete Week Eight of the Bible study. 4. Memorize this week's Scripture memory verse.
Eight	1. Greet and weigh members (15 minutes). 2. Discuss last week's challenge (5 minutes). 3. Present a wellness spotlight of your choosing (15 minutes). 4. Lead Bible study discussion (25 minutes). 5. Assign homework (2-3 minutes). 6. Prayer (5 minutes).	1. Take the physical challenge chosen by the group leader. 2. Complete Week Nine of the Bible study. 3. Memorize this week's Scripture memory verse.
Nine	1. Greet and weigh members (15 minutes). 2. Discuss last week's challenge (5 minutes). 3. Present a wellness spotlight of your choosing (15 minutes). 4. Lead Bible study discussion (25 minutes). 5. Assign homework (2-3 minutes). 6. Prayer (5 minutes).	1. Take the spiritual challenge chosen by the group leader. 2. Complete Week Ten of the Bible study. 3. Memorize this week's Scripture memory verse.

WEEK	LESSON PLAN	CHALLENGE AND HOMEWORK
Ten	1. Greet and weigh members (15 minutes). 2. Discuss last week's challenge (5 minutes). 3. Present a wellness spotlight of your choosing (15 minutes). 4. Lead Bible study discussion (25 minutes). 5. Assign homework (2-3 minutes). 6. Prayer (10 minutes).	1. Take the emotional challenge chosen by the group leader. 2. Complete Week Eleven of the Bible study. 3. Memorize this week's Scripture memory verse.
Eleven	1. Greet and weigh members (15 minutes). 2. Discuss last week's challenge (5 minutes). 3. Present a wellness spotlight of your choosing (15 minutes). 4. Lead Bible study discussion (25 minutes). 5. Assign homework (2-3 minutes). 6. Prayer (10 minutes).	1. Complete Week Twelve of the Bible study. 2. Take the mental challenge chosen by the group leader.
Twelve	1. Greet and weigh members (15 minutes). 2. Discuss last week's challenge. 3. Share member testimonies. 4. Celebrate!	1. Take the Maintenance Challenge.

Weekly Lesson Plan Form

CLASS MEETING PLAN	WEEK	DATE
Wellness Spotlight		

Wellness Worksheets	Facilitator	Materials Needed

Lesson Sequence

BIBLE STUDY

Bible Study Title	Memory Verse	Materials Needed

Lesson Sequence

Challenge and Homework

PRAYER TIME

Previous Requests	New Request

Weekly Lesson Plan Master Outline
SUBSEQUENT SESSIONS

WEEK	LESSON PLAN	CHALLENGE AND HOMEWORK
1		
2		
3		
4		
5		
6		
7		
8		
9		
10		
11		
12	Victory Celebration	

weekly challenge
ideas!

Here are a few ideas for weekly challenges to offer your group in later sessions.

EMOTIONAL CHALLENGES

- Give away or donate to charity clothes you never want to fit in again.

- Identify someone whom you have struggled to love and do an intentional act of kindness for them without them knowing.

- Make an exercise appointment with one of your fellow First Place 4 Health members this week (could also be used as a physical challenge).

- Write a letter that encourages yourself to keep going with the program. List several reasons why you should. Keep this letter for a future time when you may need some inspiration and reminder why sticking with the program is important to you.

- Reach out to someone in your First Place 4 Health group this week and learn something new about that person you can share in your meeting next week.

- Spend 15 minutes each day this week working on a project you have been putting off.

SPIRITUAL CHALLENGES

- Schedule into your week a 3-hour prayer retreat.

- Fast from television for one week.

- Meet God in a different way this week. Spend your prayer time on a nature walk and listen for Him to speak to you through His creation.

- If there is someone in your life you are having trouble loving, ask God to love that person through you.

- Go on a prayer walk this week and pray for the people in the houses you pass, the children you see playing and anyone who drives by in a car.

- Volunteer to study this week's Bible study and facilitate a discussion in next week's group meeting.

MENTAL CHALLENGES

- Learn how to do something new this week.

- Finish reading a book (and start another!).

- Learn and use five new words this week. Be prepared to share at least one word with the class and how to use it properly.

- Make it your goal to memorize a favorite chapter of Scripture over the summer.

- Create a list with two columns. In one column, list the negative self-talk you have said over and over in your mind in the past (e.g., *There is nothing I can do to improve my health*). In the other column, list positive messages that overcome the negative self-talk (e.g., *There are several things I can do to improve my health that are personalized for me*).

- Practice catching a destructive thought before you act on it, asking God to remove it from your mind.

PHYSICAL CHALLENGES

- Clean out your attic or garage this week. You'll be surprised how much physical strength it takes just to take out the trash!

- Practice standing on one foot in line at the grocery store to improve balance.

- Do as many calf-raises as possible while brushing your teeth (hold on to the bathroom sink for stability, if needed).

- Encourage your First Place 4 Health group to enter a walk/run (5K, 10K, half or full marathon) to raise money for your favorite organization.

- Try a new sport that you would have never before considered, such as golf, roller-blading or swimming.

- To improve balance, stand with both feet planted on the ground. Lift one leg and stay balanced for at least 15 seconds. Try same exercise with eyes closed. With practice, you will be able to do the exercise with eyes closed for 15 seconds, which is assessed as good balance.

MAINTENANCE CHALLENGES

- Continue filling out your Live It Tracker during the week(s) you're not in session and exchange with a fellow group-member to stay accountable. You can email, mail or set up a time to visit with that person to discuss your progress.

- Create an exercise calendar listing the activities (duration and type) you will do during the weeks you do not meet with your First Place 4 Health group.

- Choose a Bible study to work through during the session break, and work to memorize one Scripture memory verse from the study each week.

- Ask a fellow member of your group to be your prayer partner and set up a time to fellowship.

- Consider becoming a First Place 4 Health leader, inspiring others with your testimony of renewed health and weight loss.

List your ideas for weekly challenges here:

_____

_____

_____

_____

_____

_____

_____

_____

_____

six-week holiday sessions

Some groups choose to take a break over the Thanksgiving, Christmas and summer holidays. However, other groups may want to continue meeting during this time. Our six-week devotionals provide you with the option of having an abbreviated and relaxed session of First Place 4 Health if you and other members of your group feel like continuing to meet during these times.

Here are some guidelines for leading a six-week holiday session:

- Because these are shorter sessions and do not provide enough time to complete the First Place 4 Health curriculum, these sessions should only be offered to alumni.

- Continue to evaluate Live It Trackers and maintain a sense of accountability for the group. Even though the sessions may be more relaxed, First Place 4 Health basics should continue.

- Topics for wellness spotlights from *Simple Ideas for Healthy Living* may be chosen by the leader. There is no set curriculum for these shorter sessions.

- Feel free to mix things up a bit and provide a different landscape for these sessions, if desired. For example, some all-women groups have chosen in the past to discuss the Bible study while participating in craft activities and enjoying some light-hearted fellowship. Others have chosen to meet in a different member's house each week. The idea is to keep these sessions fun and flexible, as many people are pulled in many directions during these months.

Additional Resources

sharing Christ through first place 4 health

Chances are that, as a First Place 4 Health leader, you will have opportunities to share Christ with someone in your group. Below is a simple outline for sharing your faith. You can use it as a starting point in your conversations with those who are seeking God.

Spiritual transformation begins the moment we accept Jesus Christ as our Lord and Savior. Conversely, if you have not been made right with God through the saving sacrifice of Jesus, no amount of study can bring spiritual renewal. Neither can a lifetime of doing good deeds. But the Bible says that "if the Son sets you free, you will be free indeed" (John 8:36). Accepting Christ as your Lord and Savior is the essential first step in putting Him first in all things! Without the freedom that comes when you accept Jesus Christ as your personal Lord and Savior, First Place 4 Health will be just another diet and exercise program.

Do you know the God of the universe and have you invited Him into your life? If not, why not? What is stopping you? Is it unbelief that He could love you? Is it your pride in thinking that you don't really need Jesus? Could it be shame because everyone already thinks you are a Christian? Whatever it is, let it go. Let this day be the beginning of a new life in Christ.

Do you want to invite Jesus to come into your life now? It's really just a question of surrender: *Who do I want to be at the center of my life—me or Jesus Christ?*

The Bible says that we were made for God, that He seeks a relationship with each of us and that He wants us to spend eternity with Him in heaven. The bad news is that sin separates us from God and eliminates our hope of heaven. Sin is defined as missing what God wants for our lives. Think of aiming for a bull's eye and missing the mark. Sin is missing God's mark for us.

The Good News is that Jesus, God's only Son, came to Earth as a human. He willingly became our sacrifice by dying on the cross for our sins. We cannot save ourselves. Jesus has already done that for us.

Do you want to receive Christ as your Savior right now? If so, pray these words with me:

Dear God, I know I am a sinner and separated from You.
I believe You love me and that You sent Jesus to die on the cross for me.
Please forgive me of my sins and come into my life right now
and teach me how to have a new life through Jesus.
I accept You as my Savior and my Lord this day.
Amen.

Please share with someone close to you about your decision to trust Christ as your Lord and Savior!

frequently asked questions!

Over the years, we have received questions from First Place 4 Health leaders the world over. Below are some of the most popular, along with our best answers. You can discover more in-depth answers by watching the "Frequently Asked Questions" segment on the *How to Lead with Excellence* DVD. Still have questions? Visit www.firstplace4health.com to contact us or to connect with other leaders just like you!

1. What do you consider the most important quality in a leader?
    We believe the most important quality in a good leader is love.

2. What size groups work best?
    A group of 12 to 20 works well.

3. What is the format of a meeting?
    The length of each First Place 4 Health meeting is 1 hour and 15 minutes.

4. I had a person come to class who couldn't afford the materials. What should I do?
    You may offer to provide the Bible study while the person purchases the Member's Kit, or ask people in your class or church to donate toward a scholarship. We do not recommend giving full scholarships, because the person needs to invest something in order to get the most from his or her investment. We also do not recommend a payment plan unless your church is willing to absorb the cost if the member drops out.

5. I'm the only leader. I had 40 people at orientation, and they all joined. Help!
    If you find yourself with a large group and you are the only leader, we recommend dividing the group into two to four smaller teams within the large group.

6. How do you develop new leaders?

   Watch for people in your class who are doing well. Encourage them and ask for their help. It is a natural progression to go from assistant to leader, so begin looking for opportunities to involve your members in some leadership roles.

7. I've had gastric bypass surgery. Can I still lead a First Place 4 Health Group?

   Approaching weight loss with surgical methods is not a be-all, fix-all. Leaders who have had bypass surgery know that they still have to do the program—all the facets of it. It is very important for us not to judge people that come into our group, but love them.

8. How many times a year should we offer First Place 4 Health sessions?

   The program is designed as three 12-week sessions: Fall, Winter and Spring. There are also two six-week session Bible studies available to be used during summer and fall holiday seasons.

9. We don't have a lot of money. How can we publicize our program to bring in more people?

   There are many free avenues available for advertising, including:

   · Community newspapers and bulletin boards
   · Christian radio announcements
   · Flyers in physicians' waiting rooms
   · Word-of-mouth advertising
   · Members' guests at the end-of-session Victory Celebration

10. I'm the only leader at my church. How do I get encouragement?

    Ask someone in your class to be the person who encourages you and holds you accountable to your weekly weigh-ins or measurements, memory verse recitation and Live It Tracker evaluation. To ensure that you lead the best you possibly can, give adequate attention to yourself and know that you're doing yourself and your group a huge favor!

11. I have a member who loves the spiritual aspect of class (Bible study, prayer support, Scripture memory), but doesn't do the Live It plan. How should I handle this?

    Remember that First Place 4 Health is a four-sided program. God might want to work in another area in that person's life besides the physical aspect of the program. Be patient and keep encouraging him or her to embrace the program, but know that God may simply have a few more lessons to teach the person in one area before He moves on to the others.

12. I have a member who has an aversion to the scale. Does he/she have to weigh in?

    People do better when they have some form of physical accountability. Weighing is the cheapest and most convenient way to monitor a person's progress toward their weight-loss goals. Nonetheless, if you have someone with a real aversion to the scale, suggest that they weigh in at Weeks One, Six and Eleven. Or ask if they'd feel more comfortable weighing backward so that they cannot see the scale. Remember to be sensitive if you encounter a member who is afraid to weigh in. Pray for the demolishing of this stronghold in their life and wait patiently as God does His work in them (see 2 Corinthians 10:3-5).

13. I'm feeling burned out as a leader. Do you have any ideas?

The First Place 4 Health website is a rich resource for you. There are bulletin boards where you can give and receive encouragement with leaders all over the globe. Our free monthly e-newsletter is also a great source of information and practical tips for teaching and motivating your members. First Place 4 Health events are another opportunity for you to connect with leaders like you and receive support. Area meetings, workshops, national conferences, Wellness Weeks and our annual Leadership Summit are all events where leaders can come for renewed motivation, education and collaboration.

14. I have a member who monopolizes the meeting. What can I do about it?

Frequently remind the class to work at being good stewards of everyone's time and about the importance of hearing from everyone. People who monopolize meetings are usually crying out for attention. Try to give them additional attention outside of class to reduce their need to monopolize the group meetings.

15. Do alumni have to watch the *Orientation and Food Plan* DVD every session?

We feel it is important for new and returning members to watch certain foundational segments of our program each time. In subsequent sessions with mostly alumni, there is freedom beginning in Week Four and Week Five to explore other options for weekly challenges and in-class wellness spotlights. However, the repetition of fundamentals will prove effective in training up future leaders and reminding others of the essential underlying architecture of the First Place 4 Health program.

16. I have members who have lost weight and gained it back. How can I help them lose and maintain?

National statistics tell us that 95 percent of all people who lose weight will gain it back. This is discouraging news, but it is a reality that we will likely experience in First Place 4 Health from time to time. The only thing we can do is to encourage them to begin again. As they learn to give Christ first place in this area, He will help them lose weight and keep it off forever.

recommended reading
for leaders

BOOKS

Blackaby, Henry T., and Richard Blackaby. *Spiritual Leadership: The Interactive Study*. Nashville, TN: Broadman and Holman, 2006.

Larsen, Kate. *Progress Not Perfection: Your Journey Matters*. Andover, MN: Expert Publisher, 2007.

Lewis, Carole. *Stop It!* Ventura, CA: Regal Books, 2006.

Maxwell, John C. *Leadership 101: What Every Leader Needs to Know*. Nashville, TN: Thomas Nelson, Inc., 2002.

————. *The 21 Indispensable Qualities of a Leader: Becoming the Person Others Will Want to Follow*. Nashville, TN: Thomas Nelson, Inc., 2007.

————. *The Right to Lead*. Nashville, TN: Thomas Nelson, Inc., 2001.

Sanders, J. Oswald. *Spiritual Leadership: Principles of Excellence for Every Believer*. Chicago, IL: Moody Publishers, 2007.

Swanson, Jill K. *Simply Beautiful: Inside and Out*. Minneapolis, MN: Rivercity Press, Inc., 2005.

DOWNLOADS

The following articles and inventories are available to download from the Church Growth Institute's website at www.churchgrowth.org.

Fortune, Don and Katie. "Discover Your God-Given Gifts."

Gilbert, Larry. "How to Find Meaning & Fulfillment Through Understanding the Spiritual Gift Within You."

————. "Spiritual Gifts Inventory."

————. "Youth Spiritual Gifts Inventory."

Porter, Douglas. "How to Develop and Use the Gift of Administration."
——— . "How to Develop and Use the Gift of Evangelism."
——— . "How to Develop and Use the Gift of Teaching."

You can also take a free online assessment called the "Motivational Gifts Survey" at www.gifttest.org that can help you better understand how your personality and spiritual gifts help determine the kind of leader you are.

NOTES

NOTES

NOTES

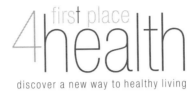

first place
4 health
discover a new way to healthy living

For more information about
First Place 4 Health,
please contact:

First Place 4 Health
7401 Katy Freeway
Houston, TX 77024
1-800-72-PLACE (727-5223)

email: info@firstplace4health.com
website: www.firstplace4health.com